NSNA Review Series

Nursing Pharmacology

Consulting Editor
Marcia E. Blicharz, Ed.D., R.N.C.
Acting Dean and Associate Professor
Trenton State College
School of Nursing
Trenton, New Jersey

Reviewers
Elizabeth A. Talbot, R.N., B.S.N.
Instructor
Weber State University
Cedar City, Utah

Joyce S. Willens, R.N., M.S.N.
Instructor
College of Nursing
Villanova University
Villanova, Pennsylvania
Doctoral Candidate
University of Maryland
Baltimore, Maryland

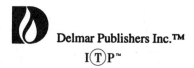

Delmar Publishers Inc.™
I(T)P™

Developed for Delmar Publishers Inc. by
    Visual Education Corporation, Princeton, New Jersey.
Publisher: David Gordon
Sponsoring Editor: Patricia Casey
Project Director: Susan J. Garver
Developmental Editor: Marguerite Kelly
Production Supervisor: Amy Davis
Proofreading Management: Christine Osborne
Word Processing: Cynthia C. Feldner
Composition: Maxson Crandall, Lisa Evans-Skopas
Cover Designer: Paul C. Uhl, DESIGNASSOCIATES
Text Designer: Circa 86

For information, address
Delmar Publishers Inc.
3 Columbia Circle
Box 15015
Albany, New York 12212

Printed in the United States of America
Published simultaneously in Canada by Nelson Canada, a
division of The Thomson Corporation

10 9 8 7 6 5 4 3 2 1

Library of Congress Cataloging-in-Publication Data

Nursing pharmacology / consulting editor, Marcia E. Blicharz;
    reviewers, Elizabeth A. Talbot, Joyce S. Willens.
        p.   cm. — (NSNA review series)
    Developed for Delmar Publishers Inc. by Visual Education
Corporation.
    ISBN 0-8273-5671-4
    1. Pharmacology—Outlines, syllabi, etc.   2. Nursing—Outlines,
syllabi, etc.   I. Blicharz, Marcia E.   II. Talbot, Elizabeth A.
III. Willens, Joyce S.   IV. Visual Education Corporation.   V. Series.
    [DNLM: 1. Pharmacology, Clinical—outlines.   2. Pharmacology,
Clinical—nurses' instruction.   3. Drug Therapy—outlines.   4. Drug
Therapy—nurses' instruction.   QV 18 N9744 1994]
RM125.N84   1994
615´.1´024613—dc20
DNLM/DLC
for Library of Congress   93-37959
                                                              CIP

Notice to the Reader

The publisher, editors, advisors, and reviewers do not warrant or guarantee any of the products described herein nor have they performed any independent analysis in connection with any of the product information contained herein. The publisher, editors, advisors, and reviewers do not assume, and each expressly disclaims, any obligation to obtain and include information other than that provided to them by the manufacturer.

The reader is expressly warned to consider and adopt all safety precautions that might be indicated by the activities described herein and to avoid all potential hazards. By following the instructions contained herein, the reader willingly assumes all risks in connection with such instructions.

The publisher, editors, advisors, and reviewers make no representations or warranties of any kind, including but not limited to the warranties of fitness for particular purpose or merchantability, nor are any such representations implied with respect to the material set forth herein, and the publisher, editors, advisors, and reviewers take no responsibility with respect to such material. The publisher, editors, advisors, and reviewers shall not be liable for any special, consequential, or exemplary damages resulting, in whole or in part, from readers' use of, or reliance upon, this material.

A conscientious effort has been made to ensure that the drug information and recommended dosages in this book are accurate and in accord with accepted standards at the time of publication. However, pharmacology is a rapidly changing science, so readers are advised, before administering any drug, to check the package insert provided by the manufacturer for the recommended dose, for contraindications for administration, and for added warnings and precautions. This recommendation is especially important for new, infrequently used, or highly toxic drugs.

CPR standards are subject to frequent change due to ongoing research. The American Heart Association can verify changing CPR standards when applicable. Recommended Schedules for Immunization are also subject to frequent change. The American Academy of Pediatrics, Committee on Infectious Diseases can verify changing recommendations.

Contents

Preface

The NSNA Review Series is a multiple-volume series designed to help nursing students review course content and prepare for course tests.

Chapter elements include:

Overview—lists the main topic headings for the chapter

Nursing Highlights—gives significant nursing care concepts relevant to the chapter

Glossary—features key terms used in the chapter that are not defined within the chapter

Enhanced Outline—consists of short, concise phrases, clauses, and sentences that summarize the main topics of course content; focuses on nursing care and the nursing process; includes the following elements:
- *Client Teaching Checklists:* shaded boxes that feature important issues to discuss with clients; designed to help students prepare client education sections of nursing care plans
- *Nurse Alerts:* shaded boxes that provide information that is of critical importance to the nurse, such as danger signs or emergency measures connected with a particular condition or situation
- *Locators:* finding aids placed across the top of the page that indicate the main outline section that is being covered on a particular 2-page spread within the context of other main section heads
- *Textbook reference aids:* boxes labeled "See text pages ___," which appear in the margin next to each main head, to be used by students to list the page numbers in their textbook that cover the material presented in that section of the outline
- *Cross references:* references to other parts of the outline, which identify the relevant section of the outline by using the numbered and lettered outline levels (e.g., "same as section I,A,1,b" or "see section II,B,3")

Chapter Tests—review and reinforce chapter material through questions in a format similar to that of the National Council Licensure Examination for Registered Nurses (NCLEX-RN); answers follow the questions and contain rationales for both correct and incorrect answers

Comprehensive Test—appears at the end of the book and includes items that review material from each chapter

1

Pharmacotherapy and the Nursing Process

OVERVIEW

I. Fundamentals of pharmacotherapy
  A. Pharmacokinetics
  B. Pharmacodynamics
  C. Factors affecting clinical response
  D. Measures of drug effectiveness
  E. Adverse reactions
  F. Drug interactions

II. The nursing process for administering and monitoring medication
  A. Nursing assessment
  B. Nursing diagnosis
  C. Nursing implementation
  D. Nursing evaluation

NURSING HIGHLIGHTS

1. In taking the client's drug history, the nurse should ask open-ended questions phrased in language appropriate to the client's socioeconomic status and educational level.
2. It is important to determine whether the client has the cognitive abilities, which can be negatively affected by disease or medication, to comply with the therapeutic regimen.
3. In questioning clients, the nurse should be aware that they may misidentify an adverse effect as an allergic response.
4. In diagnosing noncompliance, the nurse should always attempt to identify a cause, such as limited financial resources, physical or cognitive limitations in following through with therapeutic regimen, denial of health problem, or specific knowledge deficits or misunderstandings.
5. Asking clients about their socioeconomic status, educational level, lifestyle, and beliefs will help identify potential problems with compliance and important knowledge deficits.

buccal—drug administration by application to the mucous membranes of the mouth

dosage—determination of the size, number, and frequency of doses for a drug

endogenous—produced within an organism

enteral—drug administration via the alimentary tract

epidural—drug administration onto the outer membrane of the spinal cord

intrathecal—drug administration by injection into the subarachnoid space, from which it diffuses into cerebrospinal fluid

pharmacotherapeutics—study of the medicinal use of drugs, including the prevention, diagnosis, and treatment of disease

sublingual—drug administration in which medication is placed under the tongue

transdermal—drug administration through application of medication, which is systemically absorbed, to the skin

ENHANCED OUTLINE

I. Fundamentals of pharmacotherapy

See text pages

A. Pharmacokinetics: study of a drug's changes as it enters and passes through the body

1. Absorption: the drug's passage from administration site to target tissue, including its transformation from dosage form to a biologically usable form

   a) Drug routes

      (1) Enteral (oral, buccal, sublingual, or rectal, or via gastric tube): absorption mainly via small intestine but also via oral mucosa, gastric mucosa, large intestine, or rectum

      (2) Parenteral (intravenous [IV], subcutaneous [SC], intramuscular [IM], intradermal, intra-articular, intrathecal, epidural)

      (3) Topical (ointments, creams, and gels applied to skin; ophthalmic drugs; otic drugs; nasal instillations; inhalants; transdermal drug delivery system [TDDS])

   b) Mechanisms of absorption

      (1) Passive drug absorption: movement from an area of high concentration to one of low concentration by diffusion through cell membranes or pores without the expenditure of cellular energy

         (a) Only nonionized molecules can pass through cell membranes.

         (b) Weakly acidic drugs can be absorbed through the stomach, which is acidic.

         (c) Weakly alkaline drugs can be absorbed through the intestine, which is alkaline.

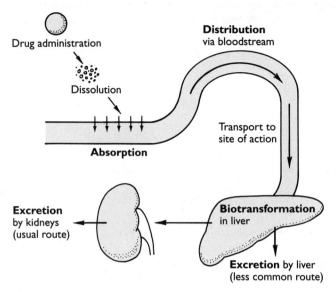

Figure 1–1
Drug Transport in the Body

(d) Small ionized molecules, such as some electrolytes, can be transported with fluids through pores in cell walls.

(e) Other compounds, such as vitamin B_{12}, are selectively transported across cell membranes by carriers.

(2) Active transport: the process by which cellular energy is used to move ionized molecules (such as electrolytes) from an area of high concentration to one of low concentration

(3) Pinocytosis: a form of phagocytosis in which the cell engulfs a drug particle and transports it actively to the inner cell in a vacuole or vesicle

c) Other factors affecting rate and amount of absorption

(1) Surface area (e.g., a client with a resected intestine will have reduced absorption of orally administered drugs)

(2) Blood flow (e.g., blood flow in intestine is increased after eating and decreased with exercise)

(3) Pain and stress (these factors decrease absorption; the cause has not been established)

(4) Gastrointestinal (GI) motility (e.g., high-fat or solid foods delay gastric emptying, retarding absorption of orally administered drugs; anticholinergics decrease intestinal motility, delaying absorption of orally administered drugs)

(5) Dosage form (e.g., sublingual tablets are absorbed more rapidly than compressed and sustained-release tablets; IM solutions are absorbed more rapidly than IM suspensions and emulsions)

(a) Rapid rate (seconds to minutes): sublingual, IV, or inhalation route

        (b) Intermediate rate (1–2 hours): oral, IM, or SC route

        (c) Slow rate (hours to days): rectal route or sustained release formulation

    (6) Drug interactions (see section I,F,2,a of this chapter)

        (a) Drug-drug interactions (e.g., tetracycline and antacid)

        (b) Drug-food interactions (e.g., tetracycline and milk)

    (7) First-pass effect: Some drugs are partially metabolized in the liver or portal vein before passing into the circulatory system.

        (a) Examples of drugs that are susceptible to a first-pass effect include dopamine, imipramine, isoproterenol, lidocaine, morphine, nitroglycerin, propranolol, reserpine, and warfarin.

        (b) The first-pass effect often explains why the recommended oral dose of an agent is far greater than the IV dose.

    (8) Drug solubility: For a drug to be absorbed, its solubility (in lipids or water) must correspond to the characteristics of the absorption site.

        (a) Only lipid-soluble cells can penetrate lipoid (fat) cells and readily cross the endothelial membrane.

        (b) Water-soluble drugs, such as penicillin, cannot pass the lipoid blood-brain barrier to enter the brain and are less able to cross the endothelial membrane.

    (9) Bioavailability: extent to which active ingredient is absorbed and transported to target tissue; variable with drug brand

    (10) Enterohepatic recycling: Some drugs, such as digoxin and digitoxin, travel intact through the biliary tract after initial absorption and are then reabsorbed into bloodstream through the intestine.

2. Distribution: the extent to which the drug passes into different tissues and fluid compartments in the body, influenced by:

  a) Drug transport: Drug is carried to site of action by albumin and other plasma proteins by plasma protein binding; this process maintains a constant ratio of bound (inactive) and unbound (active) drug.

  b) Volume distribution in body fluid compartments (e.g., blood, total body water, fat)

    (1) Water-soluble drugs have a small volume of distribution and high blood concentration because of poor penetration and high plasma protein binding.

    (2) Fat-soluble drugs have a large volume of distribution and lower blood concentration because they pass out of the vascular system into tissue more readily.

  c) Blood-brain barrier: This protective barrier allows only nonionized, unbound drug to enter brain.

3. Biotransformation (metabolism): the chemical process by which the body converts an agent from its original (parent) form to a more water-soluble form (metabolite) that can be excreted
   a) Description of the biotransformation process
      (1) A drug is usually converted by enzymes from its active form to inert metabolite(s).
      (2) Other drugs are biotransformed to both active metabolites and inert metabolites (e.g., imipramine is biotransformed to desipramine).
      (3) Some drugs are metabolized from an inactive dosage form to a more active metabolite (e.g., amitriptyline, chloral hydrate, diazepam, prednisone, propranolol).
      (4) The most common site of biotransformation is the liver, but metabolism may also occur in renal tissue, lungs, plasma, or intestinal mucosa.
   b) Types of biotransformation reactions
      (1) Synthetic or conjugation reaction: The drug or its metabolite combines with an endogenous substance, such as a carbohydrate, an alkyl group (alkylation), an acetyl group (acetylation), or a methyl group (methylation).
      (2) Nonsynthetic reaction: The drug is transformed to metabolite(s) by oxidation, reduction, or hydrolysis.
   c) Role of enzymes in biotransformation
      (1) Enzymes may increase drug's water solubility for excretion through the renal system.
      (2) Enzymes may alter drug's lipid solubility for excretion through the biliary system.
   d) Drug interactions (see section I,F,2,c of this chapter)
      (1) Some drugs may stimulate metabolism, a process called foreign induction.
      (2) Some drugs may inhibit or compete for enzyme metabolism, resulting in reduced elimination and potential toxicity.
   e) Other factors inhibiting or slowing drug metabolism
      (1) End-stage liver disease reduces metabolism of drug by liver enzymes.
      (2) Congestive heart disease reduces drug delivery to metabolic sites in the liver.
      (3) Extremes of client age limit drug metabolism (see Chapter 2, sections IV–VI).
4. Excretion: the process by which drug metabolites are eliminated from the body
   a) Drug half-life: time required for the total amount of a drug in the body to decrease by one-half; usually calculated in plasma
   b) Steady-state accumulation
      (1) If not readministered, most drugs are effectively eliminated after 5 half-lives.
      (2) If regularly readministered, most drugs achieve a steady-state concentration after 5 half-lives.

            (3) Administering a large initial dose (loading dose) followed by smaller doses (maintenance doses) is often done to reach steady-state accumulation more rapidly.

       c) Drug clearance: the rate at which drug is eliminated by the body

       d) Renal excretion: a process that takes place by glomerular filtration and/or tubular secretion

    5. Other pharmacokinetic factors affecting response to a drug

       a) Onset of action: time at which drug is sufficiently absorbed and distributed to achieve a therapeutic effect

       b) Peak concentration: highest concentration reached in blood and in target tissue

       c) Duration of action: length of time that concentration is sufficient for therapeutic effect

       d) Blood concentration level: a measure of therapeutic effect

          (1) Minimum effective concentration (MEC)

          (2) Minimum toxic concentration (MTC)

          (3) Levels that must be measured during monitoring: peak (measured 30 minutes after administration) and trough (measured 30 minutes before next dose)

B. Pharmacodynamics: mechanisms by which drugs produce changes in body tissues

    1. Nonspecific physical modification of cell environment: drug action of protective or moisturizing lotions and lubricants, stool softeners

    2. Nonspecific chemical modification of cell environment: drug action of antacids; agents that modify fluid osmolality; lipid-soluble drugs such as general anesthetics, hypnotics, and sedatives

    3. Drug-receptor interaction: interaction of drug with a specific, specialized protein, triggering a cellular response

       a) Receptors: specialized macromolecules present on cell membranes that regulate (trigger or inhibit) specific cellular activities

          (1) Changes in receptors: The number and affinity of a specific receptor type may sometimes increase (up-regulation) or decrease (down-regulation) because of the action of drugs or ligands.

          (2) Some important receptor classes

             (a) Alpha-adrenergic receptors: Stimulation produces vasoconstriction in skin and viscera.

             (b) $Beta_1$-adrenergic receptors: Stimulation increases heart rate and force of contractions.

             (c) $Beta_2$-adrenergic receptors: Stimulation produces vasodilation in skeletal and smooth muscles, especially those of the lungs and uterus.

             (d) Histamine (H_1) receptors: Stimulation produces vasodilation and contraction of smooth muscle of gut and bronchi.

        (e) Histamine (H_2) receptors: Stimulation produces secretion of hydrochloric acid in stomach and increases heart rate.

    b) Substances that bind to receptors

        (1) Ligand: an endogenous substance, such as a hormone or neuro-transmitter, that binds to and stimulates or inhibits specific receptors

        (2) Agonist: a drug that displays affinity for a receptor and enhances or stimulates its activity

        (3) Antagonist: a drug that occupies the receptor and inhibits its activity by competing with or displacing the natural agonist

    c) Mechanisms of binding to receptors: Agonists and antagonists can bind with receptors because their molecular architecture resembles that of the receptor's natural ligand.

4. Drug-enzyme interaction: binding of drug with an enzyme, causing the enzyme to catalyze a cellular biochemical reaction, increasing or decreasing the rate of that reaction

5. Nutrient-cellular interaction: drug action of vitamins and trace elements on cell function

6. Drug-subcellular interaction: drug effects on nucleic acids or other cellular components (e.g., activity of antitumor drugs on endonuclear material of malignant cells, antibiotics' activity against components of bacterial cell wall)

C. Factors affecting clinical response

  1. Diseases and disorders

    a) GI system abnormalities, including surgical resection

    b) Renal impairment from disease or aging

    c) Hepatic dysfunction, as with cirrhosis or ascites

    d) Thyroid gland abnormalities

        (1) Hypothyroidism, which slows drug metabolism

        (2) Hyperthyroidism, which speeds up drug metabolism

    e) Circulatory system abnormalities

        (1) Atherosclerosis

        (2) Peripheral vascular disease secondary to diabetes

        (3) Shock

  2. Physiologic factors

    a) Extremes of age

    b) Genetic variation in enzyme activity or enzyme deficiency (e.g., variation in acetylation rate)

    c) Muscle mass and level of body fat

    d) Circadian variations in absorption and metabolic rates

    e) Tolerance (reduced response to a drug, often due to prior exposure to that drug)

  3. Drug interactions

  4. Drug-food interactions: Some drugs bind with food and impair vitamin and mineral absorption; food alters the bioavailability of drugs absorbed through the GI tract.

D. Measures of drug effectiveness
   1. Dose-response curve: graphic representation of the therapeutic effect from administration to elimination
   2. Therapeutic index: ratio of toxic dose to therapeutic dose, calculated during animal studies while drug is in development

E. Adverse reactions: harmful, undesirable, or unexplained responses to a drug
   1. Dose-related reactions
     a) Primary reaction: overdose, an excessive therapeutic effect
     b) Secondary reaction: undesirable secondary effects (e.g., drowsiness from antihistamines)
     c) Overdose toxicity
     d) Iatrogenic drug effects (e.g., aspirin-induced GI bleeding, propranolol-induced asthma, gentamicin-induced deafness)
     e) Hypersusceptibility due to altered pharmacokinetics
   2. Sensitivity-related reactions
     a) Allergy to drug or drug metabolite
       (1) Type I—anaphylaxis: acute response of humoral system leading to cardiovascular/respiratory collapse
       (2) Type II—cytotoxic reaction: attachment of foreign antigen to target cell, which is then attacked by immune system
         (a) Client presents with fever, arthralgia, rash, splenomegaly, and lymph node enlargement.
         (b) Condition, which is usually self-limiting, occurs most commonly in clients receiving penicillin and diphtheria and tetanus antitoxin.
       (3) Type III—autoimmune reaction or complex-mediated hypersensitivity: antigen-antibody complexes carried through body by bloodstream
         (a) When complexes are deposited in tissue, they can trigger inflammatory process and tissue destruction.
         (b) Reaction is most commonly due to penicillin, phenytoin, and streptomycin.
       (4) Type IV—cell-mediated hypersensitivity: result of T-cell response
         (a) Response causes contact dermatitis.
         (b) Reaction is most commonly due to topical drugs containing benzene and phenol.
     b) Idiosyncratic response: an unexpected, abnormal response occurring in a small proportion of the population, often due to a genetic defect
   3. Drug-induced tissue and organ toxicity
     a) Dermatologic reactions: skin rashes, the most common allergic response, which can be mild or life-threatening
     b) Blood dyscrasias: uncommon but often fatal responses of hemolytic or aplastic anemia, leukopenia, agranulocytosis, or

thrombocytopenia; experienced by client as generalized weakness, fatigue, infection, or easy bruising

    c) Ocular toxicity: ranging from mild, reversible effects such as blurred vision (anticholinergics) or disturbed color vision (digitalis drugs) to permanent injury to cornea, lens, retina, or optic nerve

    d) Nephrotoxicity: arising because of kidney's role in excreting drug and large blood supply; found with aminoglycosides, analgesics, anticancer agents, and heavy metals

    e) Liver injury: occurring because of liver's role in drug biotransformation

    f) Ototoxicity: including dizziness and disturbances of balance as well as tinnitus or hearing loss; often occurring in conjunction with nephrotoxicity

    g) Sexual dysfunction: ranging from impotence to loss of libido

    h) Mutagenic effects: resulting from androgenic hormones, estrogen, anticancer drugs, caffeine, chlorpromazine, ether, griseofulvin, and colchicine

F. Drug interactions
1. IV incompatibilities: drugs that inactivate each other administered in the same IV solution (e.g., some multivitamins inactivate antibiotics by changing pH; phenytoin forms a precipitate when combined with dextrose)
2. Pharmacokinetic interactions
  a) Absorption
    (1) Gastric emptying time: Some drugs, such as anticholinergics, may prolong gastric emptying time, thereby increasing drug absorption; others (e.g., metoclopramide) may speed it up, decreasing absorption through small intestine.
    (2) pH levels: Changes in pH alter absorption rates for many drugs (e.g., antacids decrease absorption of aspirin and barbiturates but may increase absorption of amphetamines).
    (3) Complexation: Drug-drug or drug-food combinations may form nonabsorbable complexes (e.g., antacids and tetracycline).
    (4) Sequestration: Drug may be surrounded by lipoid, preventing absorption (e.g., fat-soluble vitamins and mineral oil).
  b) Distribution: Through protein and tissue binding displacement, drug A displaces drug B at binding sites, increasing unbound active drug B in serum but also increasing elimination.
  c) Biotransformation
    (1) Enzyme inducers stimulate enzyme activity in liver, increasing drug metabolism (e.g., phenobarbital).
    (2) Enzyme inhibitors decrease enzyme activity and thus increase drug effect (e.g., cimetidine).
    (3) Concurrently administered drugs that are metabolized by the same enzyme decrease the rates of metabolism and excretion for both drugs (e.g., phenytoin and isoniazid).
  d) Excretion
    (1) One drug increases or decreases renal excretion of another (e.g., diuretics reduce renal clearance of lithium).

        (2) Changes in urinary pH change drug excretion.

          (a) Alkalization increases serum levels of weak basic drugs.

          (b) Alkalization decreases levels of weak acidic drugs.

   3. Pharmacodynamic interactions

     a) Indifference: Interaction produces a combined effect equal to the single most active component of the combined drugs.

     b) Additive effect: Combined effect is equal to the sum of the effects of each drug administered alone in higher doses.

     c) Synergistic effect: Combined effect of drugs with similar therapeutic effects is greater than the sum of their effects.

     d) Potentiation effect: One drug exerts an action that is made greater by the presence of the other drug.

     e) Antagonistic effect: Combined effect is less than the effect of either drug administered alone.

See text pages

II. The nursing process for administering and monitoring medication

A. Nursing assessment

   1. Obtain drug history.

     a) Lifestyle and beliefs, including support systems, marital status, childbearing status, attitudes toward health and health care, use of health care system, activities of daily living

     b) Allergic reactions to over-the-counter (OTC) and prescription drugs and to foods

     c) Medical history, including all associated or chronic disorders

     d) All prescription and OTC drugs

        (1) Reason for use

        (2) Client's knowledge base about drug

        (3) Frequency or dosage

        (4) Effectiveness and reactions

     e) Habits

        (1) Dietary

        (2) Exercise

        (3) Recreational drug use, including alcohol, tobacco, and stimulants such as caffeine, as well as illegal drugs, with frequency and amount used

     f) Sensory deficits, especially those affecting ability to self-administer

     g) Socioeconomic status, including age, educational level, occupation, and health insurance coverage

   2. Determine baseline measurements needed to monitor safety and efficacy of drug regimen (e.g., creatinine clearance, complete blood count, thyroid function tests, liver function tests).

B. Nursing diagnosis
   1. Main drug-specific nursing diagnoses
      a) Knowledge deficit related to drug therapy, as evidenced by client's:
         (1) Statement of misconception
         (2) Request for information
         (3) Errors in following instructions
         (4) Signs of cognitive impairment
      b) Noncompliance related to drug therapy, as evidenced by:
         (1) Acknowledgment of failure to follow regimen by client or informed observer
         (2) Failure on objective tests
         (3) Development of complications
         (4) Exacerbation of symptoms
         (5) Failure to improve or progress
         (6) Failure to keep appointments
   2. Examples of other drug-specific nursing diagnoses
      a) High risk for injury related to anticoagulant therapy
      b) Sexual dysfunction related to antihypertensive medication
      c) Altered nutrition, less than body requirements, related to nausea and anorexia caused by chemotherapy
      d) Altered urinary elimination related to urinary retention caused by antihistamine therapy
      e) Fluid volume excess related to edema caused by steroid therapy
      f) Sleep pattern disturbance related to insomnia caused by buspirone
      g) Altered role performance related to benzodiazepine dependence
      h) Anxiety related to cosmetic changes caused by carbamazepine

C. Nursing implementation
   1. Administer medication as prescribed (see also Chapter 2, section III).
   2. Monitor client for therapeutic effect.
   3. Evaluate serum drug level and results of relevant laboratory tests.
   4. Monitor client for adverse effects, toxicity, and drug interactions; notify physician if any are observed.
   5. Teach client about medication and importance of compliance; include family members as appropriate (see also Chapter 2, section VII).
   6. Monitor client compliance by the following means:
      a) Physiologic measurements, such as serum or urine drug level
      b) Judgment by attending physician or other health team member
      c) Client self-report
      d) Pill counts
      e) Direct observation

D. Nursing evaluation—sample types
   1. Client obtains expected effects of prescribed drug.
   2. Client avoids adverse effects and drug interactions.
   3. Client demonstrates an understanding of his/her medication as taught, including reason for taking, contraindications, and necessary self-administration.
   4. Client complies with the prescribed therapeutic regimen.

1. Crushing an enteric-coated tablet before administering it to a client is most likely to result in:

   a. Increased risk of drug toxicity.
   b. The need to take the drug with meals.
   c. Impaired intestinal absorption of the drug.
   d. Undesirable interactions between the drug and gastric contents.

2. The nurse would expect to see drug effects most rapidly after which route of administration?

   a. Oral capsules
   b. Intramuscular injection
   c. Rectal suppository
   d. Metered dose inhaler

3. Morphine has a large hepatic first-pass effect. Based on this information, the nurse should anticipate which of the following when a client is switched from intramuscular (IM) to oral (PO) morphine?

   a. The PO dose will be much larger than the IM dose.
   b. The PO dose will be much smaller than the IM dose.
   c. The PO dose will be equal to the IM dose.
   d. Loading doses must be given before routine PO dosing begins.

4. Which of the following laboratory results would indicate that a client is at an unusually high risk for a toxic reaction to a highly protein-bound drug?

   a. Serum protein 9.1 g/dl (normal 6.6 to 7.9 g/dl)
   b. Serum calcium 12.1 mg/dl (normal 8.9 to 10.1 mg/dl)
   c. Serum albumin 2.1 g/dl (normal 3.3 to 4.5 g/dl)
   d. Serum glucose 180 mg/dl (normal 70 to 110 mg/dl)

5. Ms. Ephraim began taking fluoxetine (Prozac) for depression 3 days ago. She tells the nurse, "I have taken every pill the way I was told, but I don't feel any better." Which is the most appropriate action for the nurse to take?

   a. Notify the physician that fluoxetine is not having the desired therapeutic effect.
   b. Assess Ms. Ephraim for factors that would impair absorption of fluoxetine.
   c. Explain that it will take at least 10 days for the full therapeutic effect of fluoxetine to appear.
   d. Check Ms. Ephraim's serum protein levels for excessive protein binding of fluoxetine.

6. When evaluating whether a client is at high risk for drug cumulation, it is most important for the nurse to check the results of which of the following tests?

   a. Serum lipids
   b. Serum albumin
   c. Blood urea nitrogen (BUN)
   d. Liver enzymes

7. A drug that binds to a receptor and initiates a response is called a(n):

   a. Agonist.
   b. Competitive antagonist.
   c. Noncompetitive antagonist.
   d. Ligand.

8. Clients often interpret distressing side effects as allergic responses to drugs. Which of the following descriptions by a client is most likely to reflect a drug side effect rather than an allergic reaction?

   a. "I felt like my throat was closing and I couldn't breathe."
   b. "I felt nauseated every time I took a pill and sometimes I vomited."
   c. "I got a fever and my joints were achy."
   d. "I got a rash that looked like little blisters and was itchy."

9. An organ that is commonly affected by drug toxicities is the:

   a. Bone marrow.
   b. Heart.
   c. Brain.
   d. Kidney.

10. The drug cimetidine blocks gastric acid secretion, raising the pH of the stomach. In monitoring the effects of other medications taken by a client who receives cimetidine, it would be most important for the nurse to assess for:

    a. Increased side effects of weakly acidic drugs.
    b. Decreased therapeutic effects of weakly acidic drugs.
    c. Decreased therapeutic effects of weakly alkaline drugs.
    d. Increased gastric distress caused by all types of drugs.

11. John has been taking theophylline to control asthma for 2 years. Theophylline is inactivated by the microsomal enzymes in the liver. John is now scheduled to begin taking rifampin, which induces microsomal enzymes. Based on this information, the nurse should observe John closely for:

    a. Theophylline toxicity.
    b. Rifampin toxicity.
    c. An increase in asthma symptoms.
    d. Hepatotoxicity.

12. Which of the following statements by a client would support a nursing diagnosis of noncompliance with drug therapy?

    a. "I don't understand why I have to keep taking the pills when I'm not coughing any more."
    b. "I can't see the lines on the syringe very well, but I can tell the dose is right by how far I pull up the plunger."
    c. "My pulse was only 50, so I didn't take my digoxin today."
    d. "When I get headaches I know my blood pressure is up, so I take the medicine for a few days."

ANSWERS

1. **Correct answer is d.** Enteric coatings dissolve in the alkaline environment of the intestine, preventing contact between the drug and gastric contents when those contents might inactivate or alter the drug.

   a. Crushing enteric-coated medications would not increase absorption, so increased toxicity is unlikely. Toxicity is a concern when sustained-release formulations are crushed.
   b. The enteric-coated medication is probably being used because taking the drug with food would not provide adequate protection from drug-induced gastric irritation. Deciding to eliminate the protection of the enteric coating and administer the drug with meals would not be a nursing measure.
   c. Crushing medications generally speeds absorption but does not alter the total amount of drug absorbed.

2. **Correct answer is d.** Drugs are most rapidly absorbed via intravenous, inhalation, and sublingual routes, so drug effects would appear most quickly (within minutes) when one of these routes is used.

   a. Oral medications are absorbed at an intermediate rate, so effects would appear over 1 to 2 hours.
   b. Although the IM route provides more rapid absorption than the oral route, parenteral routes have an intermediate rate of absorption.
   c. The rectal route has a slow rate of absorption, so effects appear over several hours

3. **Correct answer is a.** Because the portal circulation will carry all absorbed morphine from an oral dose through the liver before it enters general circulation, much of the dose will be inactivated before it reaches other tissues. Oral doses must be large enough that the portion that escapes first-pass inactivation is adequate for therapeutic effect. Parenteral doses are not affected by hepatic first-pass effects.

b. Smaller oral doses would be insufficient for therapeutic effect.

c. Since part of the oral dose will be inactivated by the hepatic first-pass effect, the same dose would probably be inadequate to produce therapeutic blood levels.

d. Loading doses are used to saturate tissue binding sites. Because hepatic first-pass effects involve inactivation of the drug rather than binding to tissues, loading doses would not be helpful.

4. **Correct answer is c.** A decrease in available protein binding sites leaves more unbound (i.e., active) drug available, increasing the risk of toxicity. Albumin, the major serum protein, is most often used to evaluate protein binding site availability.

   a. An increase in available serum proteins to bind the drug would result in an unexpectedly large portion of inactivated drug.

   b. Calcium in the blood does not bind drugs, nor does it alter the rate of protein binding.

   d. Because glucose has no effect on protein binding, it would not be useful in evaluating the toxic potential of protein-bound drugs.

5. **Correct answer is c.** Fluoxetine has a half-life of 48 hours. Since it takes 5 half-lives to achieve the complete therapeutic effect of a drug, full effects of fluoxetine are not expected for 10 days. The nurse should help the client change her unrealistic expectation of immediate results.

   a. Notifying the physician would be premature, since full therapeutic effect is not yet anticipated.

   b. Although a problem with absorption is possible, this assessment is premature.

   d. Serum albumin would provide information about protein binding. Because there is no indication that fluoxetine is highly protein bound, this action is not appropriate.

6. **Correct answer is c.** Since most drugs are excreted by the kidneys, evaluation of renal function is important in evaluating the risk of cumulation. BUN, usually in combination with serum creatinine, is used to determine renal function.

   a. Serum lipids do not affect drug levels. Drugs that bind to lipids become attached to adipose tissues in the body, not to lipids in the blood.

   b. Serum albumin predicts the degree of protein binding, which does not affect drug excretion. Thus it is not useful in evaluating the risk of cumulation.

   d. Liver enzymes are used to determine liver disease or damage, which would affect biotransformation. Biotransformation does affect excretion of certain drugs. However, kidney function has a more direct impact and applies to a majority of drugs, so it is a better screening tool for cumulation.

7. **Correct answer is a.** An agonist has an affinity for a receptor and, upon binding, initiates the receptor's expected function.

   b. An antagonist binds to a receptor and prevents the ligand from binding to it, so that the drug does not initiate the receptor's usual function. A competitive antagonist can be displaced from some receptors when the concentration of the ligand is increased.

   c. A noncompetitive antagonist is not displaced from receptors, whatever the ligand's concentration. As an antagonist, it prevents the receptor's usual function.

   d. A ligand is an endogenous substance, such as a hormone or neurotransmitter, that binds to the receptor to produce the expected function.

8. **Correct answer is b.** Nausea is a common side effect of medications, usually related to irritation of the stomach lining by a foreign substance. Taking more fluid or a snack with the medication usually controls this effect.

a. The sensation that the throat is closing and an inability to breathe are symptoms of a type I (anaphylactic) response.
c. Fever and painful joints are symptoms of a type II (cytotoxic) reaction.
d. Development of an itchy rash with blisters is a symptom of a type IV (cell-mediated hypersensitivity) response.

9. **Correct answer is d.** Drug toxicities usually affect the organs that have the most contact with drugs: the liver, where most drugs are metabolized, and the kidneys, where most drugs are excreted.

   a. Bone marrow toxicity, which produces blood dyscrasias, is very serious but rare.
   b. Although drugs in circulating blood pass through the heart, few have a specific affinity for heart tissue. Thus, cardiac toxicity is uncommon.
   c. Because the blood-brain barrier protects the brain from contact with many drugs, it is not a common site of drug toxicity.

10. **Correct answer is b.** Normally, weakly acidic drugs are absorbed well from the strongly acid environment of the stomach. Increasing gastric pH (i.e., lessening acidity) will reduce absorption of these drugs, decreasing their therapeutic effects.

    a. Since absorption of acidic drugs would probably be decreased, there would be no effect on side effects or a decreased likelihood of side effects.
    c. Weakly alkaline drugs are normally absorbed from the alkaline environment of the small intestine. Reducing gastric acidity would not change intestinal alkalinity.
    d. Drug-induced gastric distress is usually caused by irritation of the gastric lining. Gastric acid might potentiate this distress. If reduced acidity had any effect, it would probably be to reduce gastric distress.

11. **Correct answer is c.** When a drug induces microsomal enzymes, metabolism of all drugs affected by these enzymes is speeded up. This process may decrease blood levels and therapeutic effect of a drug. A client taking theophylline might experience increased asthma symptoms.

    a. Theophylline toxicity would occur if blood levels rose. This might occur if John had been taking both drugs and the rifampin were discontinued.
    b. Since theophylline does not induce microsomal enzymes, it would not alter rifampin's rate of metabolism.
    d. Induction of microsomal enzymes improves the liver's detoxification function and does not cause liver damage.

12. **Correct answer is d.** Antihypertensive medications must be taken regularly to be effective. Taking them only in response to symptoms will not control high blood pressure, which is often asymptomatic. This client is acknowledging failure to follow the prescribed regimen.

    a. The client who cannot see the point of taking medication when the presenting problem appears to have been resolved is requesting information, which is an indicator for the diagnosis "knowledge deficit."
    b. The client who cannot see the lines on a syringe is reporting a sensory deficit that may interfere with the prescribed therapy. Since this method may result in inaccurate dosage with dangerous effects, an appropriate nursing diagnosis would be "high risk for injury related to inaccuracy in measuring insulin dosage."
    c. The client who skips doses of digoxin because of a low pulse rate is acting correctly.

2

Issues of Drug Safety and Efficacy

VII. Teaching clients about their medication and promoting client compliance
  A. Nursing assessment criteria
  B. Methods of making nursing diagnoses
  C. Nursing intervention procedures
  D. Methods of evaluating compliance at follow-up

NURSING HIGHLIGHTS

1. In dealing with children, the nurse should give a simple, age-appropriate explanation of the procedure just before performing it.
2. Before administering a drug intravenously or intramuscularly, the nurse should let the child know that it is all right to cry but that he/she needs to hold still.
3. The nurse should warn the child before a painful procedure, praise all attempts to cooperate, and never try to embarrass the child for poor self-control.
4. If a parent is not present, the nurse should comfort the infant or child after a painful procedure.
5. Whenever possible, the nurse should provide the older child with options before performing a procedure so that he/she feels more in control.
6. The nurse should educate pregnant clients and women attempting to become pregnant about the risk of using medication, including over-the-counter (OTC) drugs, and warn them never to self-medicate during pregnancy.
7. When communicating with an elderly client with hearing loss, the nurse should speak slowly and pitch the voice low for better comprehension.
8. The nurse should evaluate elderly clients' physical and cognitive abilities to self-administer medication. Can they see well enough to read labels and tell their pills apart? Can they open their medication containers? Can they follow instructions about taking their medicine with meals or at a set time before or after meals?
9. A drug schedule or calendar on which the client checks off or scratches off medications as they are taken may help an elderly person remember to take medications.
10. Because elderly clients may borrow medications from a friend or relative with similar symptoms, the nurse should ask specifically about this practice when taking the drug history.
11. The nurse should be especially alert to possible drug interactions in the elderly, who often take multiple drugs prescribed by different physicians.

GLOSSARY

bioequivalence—relationship between two or more formulations of the same drug that have virtually identical pharmacologic properties, including the same amounts of active ingredient(s) and the same levels of absorption into the bloodstream

generic drug—a drug formulation sold after the period of patent protection for the original name-brand formulation has expired

legend drug—a drug that is required to bear the warning: "Caution: Federal law prohibits dispensing without a prescription." This category includes drugs given by injection, habit-forming drugs, those that must be administered under the supervision of a physician or dentist, and investigational drugs.

teratogen—an agent or environmental factor that causes fetal defects

ENHANCED OUTLINE

See text pages

I. U.S. drug legislation

A. Pure Food and Drug Act (1906)
   1. Required labeling for presence of 11 identified dangerous or addictive ingredients
   2. Prohibited false and misleading claims made on packaging (but not in other advertising materials)
   3. Sherley Amendment (1912) prohibited false therapeutic claims

B. Harrison Narcotic Act (1914)
   1. Attempted to curb drug addiction and dependence for the first time
   2. Established "narcotic" as a legal term

C. Food, Drug, and Cosmetic Act (1938)
   1. Required safety studies before a new drug could be marketed
   2. Required drug labels to be accurate and complete

D. Durham-Humphrey Amendment (1952)
   1. Required legend drugs to be dispensable only by prescription
   2. Required legend drug prescriptions to be refillable only with physician authorization
   3. Recognized class of OTC drugs not requiring a prescription

E. Kefauver-Harris Amendment (1962)
   1. Required proof of both safety and efficacy before a drug could be approved for use
   2. Established drug testing methods
   3. Required that all drugs introduced from 1936 to 1962 be rated for effectiveness and ineffective drugs be withdrawn from the market
   4. Gained strong support in the wake of the thalidomide tragedy in Europe

F. Controlled Substances Act of 1970
   1. Designed to curb drug abuse
   2. Categorized drugs by their potential for abuse (see section II of this chapter)

G. Drug Regulation Reform Act of 1978
   1. Streamlined the drug investigation process
   2. Allowed for earlier release of new drugs to the public

H. Drug Price Competition and Patent Term Restoration Act of 1984
   1. Allowed marketing of generic drugs after proof of bioequivalence
   2. Extended patent protection on new drugs

II. Controlled substances

See text pages _____

A. Schedule I drugs (e.g., heroin, marijuana, LSD, mescaline)
   1. High abuse potential—may lead to severe dependence
   2. No accepted medical use—available only for research purposes

B. Schedule II drugs (e.g., opium, morphine, codeine, cocaine, methadone, amphetamine)
   1. High abuse potential—may lead to severe physical and/or psychologic dependence
   2. Accepted medical uses—written prescription required, no refills permitted

C. Schedule III drugs (e.g., preparations containing limited codeine or morphine; nonnarcotic derivatives of barbituric acid)
   1. Less abuse potential than Schedule I and II drugs—may lead to moderate/low physical dependence or high psychologic dependence
   2. Accepted medical uses—written or oral prescription required, with refills limited to 5

D. Schedule IV drugs (e.g., barbital, phenobarbital, chloral hydrate, meprobamate)
   1. Less abuse potential than Schedule III drugs—may lead to limited physical or psychologic dependence
   2. Accepted medical uses—written or oral prescription required, with refills limited to 5

E. Schedule V drugs (e.g., preparations containing limited opioids)
   1. Less abuse potential than Schedule IV drugs—may lead to limited physical or psychologic dependence
   2. Accepted medical uses—prescription may be required, depending on state law

III. The nurse's responsibilities

See text pages _____

A. Liability
   1. The nurse's role in administering and even prescribing medication is expanding.
   2. Along with the pharmacist and the physician, the nurse is legally responsible for safe and therapeutically effective drug administration.
   3. Nurses are liable for their actions and omissions as well as for duties they delegate to others.

B. The Five Rights
 1. The right medication
 2. The right client
 3. The right dosage
 4. The right form, route, and technique
 5. The right time

C. Precautions and techniques for drug administration
 1. For all medication
     a) Identify the client by name and by checking the identification bracelet. Compare the medication sheet with the bracelet. Verify the Five Rights.
     b) State the name and purpose of the medication to the client.
     c) Do not leave medication with client unless specifically ordered.
 2. Enteral medication
     a) Never divide unscored tablets, enteric-coated tablets, or capsules.
     b) Shake the correct number of pills or capsules into the lid, then into the souffle cup; do not touch them directly.
     c) Position client for safe administration, avoiding aspiration and enhancing absorption.
     d) Stay with client until all the medication has been swallowed with adequate fluid.
     e) Utilize liquid formulations as often as possible when administering medication to clients with gastric tubes.
 3. Parenteral medication
     a) Know and use the correct type of needle and syringe for every injection type.
     b) Check with pharmacist or another resource about drug compatibility before mixing medications in the same syringe.
     c) Rotate subcutaneous (SC) injection sites according to pattern.
     d) Be able to identify the most common intramuscular (IM) sites, including ventrogluteal, dorsogluteal, deltoid, vastus lateralis, and rectus femoris; inappropriate sites may cause lasting injury.
     e) Rotate IM sites to avoid muscle damage.

D. Nursing principles for safe and effective drug administration
 1. Always verify the Five Rights.
 2. Wash hands between clients and before administering medication.
 3. Chart drug administration only after the drug has been given, never before.
 4. Never leave the medication tray or cart unattended.
 5. Check the discontinuation date on the medication sheet before administering drugs to be sure they are given only for the prescribed time period.
 6. Chart observed therapeutic and adverse drug effects accurately and fully.
 7. Inform the prescribing physician of any observed adverse effects.

8. Check the client history for allergies and potential drug interactions before administering a newly ordered drug.
9. Question drug orders that are unclear, that appear to contain errors, or that have a potential to harm.
10. Observe all proper accounting procedures in dispensing controlled substances.
11. Take the following actions if an error occurs:
    a) Immediately notify the nursing supervisor, the prescribing physician, and the pharmacist.
    b) Assess the client's condition and provide any necessary care.

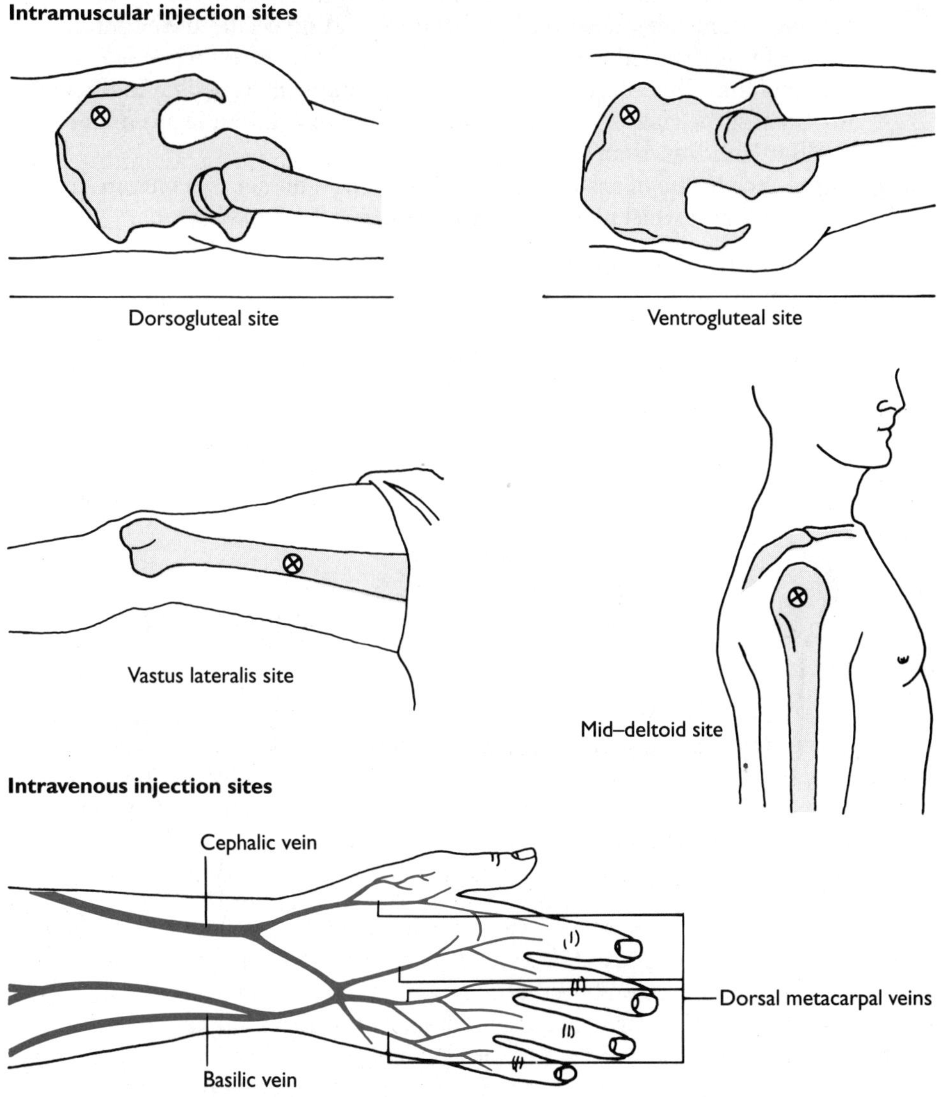

Intramuscular injection sites

Dorsogluteal site

Ventrogluteal site

Vastus lateralis site

Mid–deltoid site

Intravenous injection sites

Cephalic vein

Dorsal metacarpal veins

Basilic vein

Figure 2–1
Intramuscular and Intravenous Injection Sites

See text pages
_____

IV. The pediatric client—differences from adult clients

A. Pharmacokinetic differences
1. Absorption: Gastric emptying time is variable; gastric pH is higher; most medications are administered when stomach is empty; milk may deactivate some oral medications.
2. Distribution: Total fluid volume is higher in infants, diluting water-soluble drugs; decreased plasma protein binding occurs in the infant, intensifying drug effects.
3. Metabolism: The infant's immature liver makes metabolism inefficient, increasing the risk of toxicity; metabolism by oxidation is often more rapid in children than in adults.
4. Excretion: Kidneys are immature at birth and do not concentrate urine at adult levels until about 3 months of age.

B. Pharmacodynamic differences
1. Mechanism of action is the same at all ages, but organ immaturity will affect the response.
2. Receptor sensitivity varies in infants and young children.

C. Dosage calculations
1. The range per kilogram of body weight can be determined.
2. Body surface area can be calculated by using a nomogram.

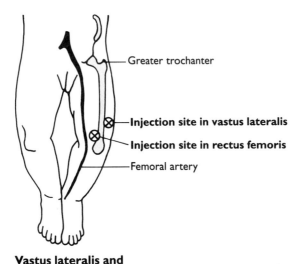

Vastus lateralis and rectus femoris sites

Figure 2–2
IM Injection Sites Preferred for Infants and Toddlers

D. Oral administration techniques
   1. For a small child or infant, use a syringe with a Brody tip to administer the dose in drops into the side of the mouth.
   2. Do not attempt to administer medication in formula; medication can be made more palatable by adding a small amount of syrup.

E. Intramuscular administration techniques
   1. Use the smallest-gauge needle suitable for the medication (see Nurse Alert, "Intramuscular Injections and Emboli").
   2. It is usually best to use the vastus lateralis and rectus femoris in infants and toddlers.
   3. Dorsogluteal and ventrogluteal sites can be used in children who have been walking for at least 1 year.

F. Intravenous administration techniques
   1. A more lateral intravenous (IV) catheter site is preferred because it reduces the chances of dislodging the needle.
   2. A padded board should be used to secure the foot or hand in which the catheter has been inserted.
   3. Because infants, small children, and children with compromised cardiovascular status are susceptible to fluid overload:
      a) Use a volume control set.
      b) Limit fluid to 2 hours' worth at a time.
   4. Because position changes, crying, and restraints can all impede flow, check client regularly.

G. Topical administration precautions
   1. Be aware that the thin epidermis and large body-surface area of infants and small children increase absorption and add to the risk of toxicity, especially with topical corticosteroids.
   2. Apply topical medication as sparingly as possible.

V. The pregnant or lactating client—differences from other adult clients

A. Pharmacokinetic differences

┌─────────────────┐
│ See text pages │
│ ───────────── │
└─────────────────┘

   1. Absorption: GI changes slow absorption of oral drugs; peripheral vasodilation may speed absorption of parenterally administered drugs (see Nurse Alert, "Pregnancy and Gastrointestinal Problems").
   2. Distribution: Fluid volume increases; hormonal competition for plasma binding increases the active drug fraction.

      3. Metabolism: Placenta is metabolically active and can change drug metabolism, increasing or decreasing metabolite potency.

      4. Excretion: Increased renal plasma flow accelerates the elimination of some drugs.

B. Fetal pharmacokinetics

      1. Knowledge of most drugs' effects on the fetus is limited.

      2. Fetal circulation may influence drug distribution and binding.

      3. The fetus has a slower drug clearance than the adult.

      4. The unborn's susceptibility to adverse effects is greatest in first trimester, when organs are developing (see Nurse Alert, "Common Teratogens").

      5. Intrauterine growth retardation may result from exposure to a teratogenic drug later in pregnancy.

      6. Teratogenesis can result from several different mechanisms.

         a) Drugs may alter maternal tissue, affecting the fetus indirectly.

         b) Drugs may alter nutrient transport or placental metabolism, impairing fetal nutrition.

         c) Drugs may exert a direct effect on the embryonic cells, causing specific abnormalities.

         d) Drugs may have long-delayed effects on the health and behavior of the child.

C. Drugs affecting lactation

      1. Anesthetics, sedatives, and alcohol may affect the milk ejection reflex.

      2. Thiazide diuretics may suppress lactation.

      3. Hormones may reduce milk production and milk protein.

      4. Antipsychotics may cause galactorrhea.

      5. Nicotine may reduce milk production.

      6. Bromocriptine may suppress lactation.

! NURSE *ALERT* !

Pregnancy and Gastrointestinal Problems

Pregnancy often is accompanied by heartburn, nausea, and constipation, but many of the OTC products commonly used for these complaints have not been approved for use in pregnancy.

- Few data are available on antacids' effects on the fetus. Sodium bicarbonate and magnesium trisilicate should not be used.
- A number of antinausea agents, including prochlorperazine maleate (Compazine), diphenhydramine hydrochloride (Benadryl), and trimethobenzamide hydrochloride (Tigan) have been linked with birth defects.
- Some laxatives (castor oil, hyperosmotic saline cathartics, lubricants) are not safe or not recommended for use during pregnancy.

D. Drugs contraindicated for breastfeeding mothers
   1. Methotrexate, cyclophosphamide, cyclosporine, and doxorubicin may cause immune system suppression and have a possible role in carcinogenesis and unknown effects on growth.
   2. Cimetidine concentrates in milk, suppresses gastric acidity, stimulates the central nervous system (CNS), and inhibits drug metabolism.
   3. Ergotamine may cause vomiting, diarrhea, and seizures.
   4. Gold salts may cause rash and kidney and liver inflammation.
   5. Methimazole may affect thyroid function.
   6. Lithium may lead to significant blood levels of that agent in the infant.
   7. Chloramphenicol may cause bone marrow depression.

VI. The geriatric client—differences from younger adult clients

See text pages
_____

A. Pharmacokinetic differences
   1. Absorption: Age slows but does not reduce absorption.
   2. Distribution: Reduced albumin production in the liver causes a reduction in plasma protein binding; total body mass declines and total body water decreases with the relative increase of body fat, changing distribution patterns.
      a) Fat-soluble drugs (e.g., diazepam) have an increased volume of distribution and a prolonged half-life.
      b) Water-soluble drugs (e.g., gentamicin) have a decreased volume of distribution and a higher serum concentration.
   3. Metabolism: The liver's efficiency in metabolizing drugs declines with age; one factor is the decline in hepatic circulation.
   4. Excretion: Age-related decline in renal function is not always heralded by increased serum creatine levels; the risk of nephrotoxicity (e.g., with aminoglycosides) is greater in the elderly.

B. Pharmacodynamic differences
   1. Decline in the sensitivity of many types of receptors causes a diminished response to various drugs.
   2. Reduction in the number of beta-adrenergic receptors increases the risk of toxicity from beta-blockers.

3. Reduction in neurotransmitters, especially dopamine and acetylcholine, occurs.

C. Drug-related organ system changes

1. Central nervous system
   a) Lipid-soluble drugs accumulate.
   b) The elderly have a heightened sensitivity to CNS depressants (e.g., barbiturates and general anesthetics).
   c) Cimetidine has CNS adverse effects (e.g., confusion, disorientation) and reduces metabolism and excretions of some drugs, including benzodiazepines.

2. Cardiovascular system
   a) Blood vessel elasticity declines, decreasing flow to some parts of the body.
   b) Renal and hepatic circulation may be reduced, slowing drug metabolism and excretion.
   c) Diuretics can cause severe fluid volume deficit, resulting in reduced cardiac output and hypotension.
   d) Antihypertensives can also reduce cardiac output and blood pressure.
   e) Orthostatic hypotension resulting from diuretics, antihypertensives, or anticholinergics can contribute to neuropathy, organic brain disease, or dehydration.

3. Respiratory system
   a) Capacity and flow rate decrease.
   b) Sensitivity to respiratory depressants (e.g., narcotics and barbiturates) increases.

4. Gastrointestinal (GI) system
   a) GI motility and activity are reduced.
   b) Sensitivity to GI effects of anticholinergics increases.

5. Urinary system
   a) Renal function, particularly glomerular filtration, declines progressively.
   b) Digoxin, aminoglycosides, nitrofurantoin, and other drugs excreted primarily by glomerular filtration should be given in reduced dosages.
   c) Nonsteroidal anti-inflammatory drugs (NSAIDs) can contribute to renal dysfunction by reducing renal prostaglandin production.
   d) Digitalis toxicity is more likely to occur.

6. Endocrine system
   a) Blood glucose tends to rise with age; however, hypoglycemia also occurs, with more subtle signs and symptoms than in the young.
   b) Blood glucose levels must be monitored in elderly clients receiving either hyperglycemic or hypoglycemic agents.

7. Musculoskeletal system
   a) Beta-carotene and cholecalciferol can change bone composition, increasing the risk of fracture.
   b) Furosemide depletes serum calcium and increases the risk of osteoporosis, especially in women.
   c) Sedatives, hypnotics, and other drugs causing muscle weakness can increase the risk of falls.

VII. Teaching clients about their medication and promoting client compliance

See text pages

_____

A. Nursing assessment criteria
   1. Assess client's educational level, reading and vocabulary levels, and cognitive abilities.
   2. Assess client's present knowledge base.
   3. Assess presence of supportive family members, as well as their educational level and knowledge base.
   4. Assess client's physical and emotional readiness to learn.
      a) The client needs time for adjustment after surgery or diagnosis of a serious illness.
      b) Panic, severe anxiety, or depression will interfere with learning.
   5. Note the existence of a cultural background that might affect client's outlook on present state of health and treatment plan.

B. Methods of making nursing diagnoses
   1. Identify specific information deficits concerning:
      a) Disorder or condition.
      b) Medication and health care regimen.
      c) Potential for injury associated with therapeutic regimen.
      d) Diet and exercise.
   2. Identify skills needed for self-care and compliance (e.g., ability to self-inject insulin).
   3. Identify psychologic factors interfering with compliance, e.g., denial of illness, low self-esteem, fear or anxiety (see Nurse Alert, "Predictors of Noncompliance").

! NURSE *ALERT* !

Predictors of Noncompliance

Attitudes, traits, and behaviors that suggest that a client is at risk for noncompliance:
- Low self-esteem
- Limited coping skills
- Denial of the seriousness of the disorder
- Failure to understand treatment goals
- Dissatisfaction with present or past medical care
- Negative opinions about the health care team

C. Nursing intervention procedures
  1. Formulate a teaching plan.
    a) Approaches and materials to be used (e.g., individual and group discussions, videotapes, pamphlets)
    b) Method of evaluation to be used (e.g., discussion, demonstration, written or oral quizzes)
    c) Best ways to involve client's family in the teaching process
  2. Establish the major points to be covered.
    a) Purpose of medication
    b) Length of time medication will be needed, including importance of refilling prescription to cover entire time
    c) How and when to take medication
    d) How to tell that the medication is effective
    e) Possible and probable side effects and what to do about them
    f) Drug-drug and drug-food interactions
    g) Signs and symptoms to report to physician
    h) What to do when one or more doses are missed
    i) Proper storage of medication
    j) Required follow-up

D. Methods of evaluating compliance at follow-up: questions to ask the client
  1. How do you take your medication?
  2. How often do you take it?
  3. How do you feel it is helping you?
  4. What side effects are you having?
  5. How much do the side effects bother you?
  6. What other problems are you experiencing?

```
Medication card

Client's name _____

Reason _____

Medication _____

How to take _____

Possible problems _____

What to do _____

_____

_____
Do not stop taking this medication without talking to your doctor first.
```

Figure 2–3
Sample Medication Information Card

1. Under the terms of the Drug Price Competition and Patent Term Restoration Act of 1984, a generic medication may be substituted for a brand-name drug if:
   a. The physician's approval for the substitution is obtained.
   b. Bioequivalence of the generic and brand-name drugs has been shown through research.
   c. The generic drug is identical to the brand-name drug.
   d. The client requests the substitution to reduce medication costs.

2. Under the Controlled Substances Act of 1970, Schedule II drugs may be dispensed:
   a. Over the counter unless prohibited by state law.
   b. With a written or oral prescription.
   c. Only with a written prescription.
   d. Only if the client is a subject in an approved research study.

3. All of the following orders appear on a medication order sheet that has the client's name imprinted on it and is signed by the physician. Which one contains all information necessary to allow the nurse to administer the drug correctly?
   a. Digoxin 0.25 mg PO daily
   b. Septra ii QID PO
   c. Theo-Dur 200 mg TID
   d. Robitussin i tsp PO PRN

4. When the nurse arrives to administer 10:00 A.M. medications to Mr. Johnson, he is taking a shower. Mr. Johnson says, "Just leave them on my bedside table. I'll take them when I come out." What should the nurse do?
   a. Leave the medications on the bedside table and chart that they were administered.
   b. Leave the medications on the bedside table and ask Mr. Johnson to inform the nurse when he has taken them.
   c. Return the pills to their original containers and pour them again when Mr. Johnson is ready to take them.
   d. Label the cup containing the pills with Mr. Johnson's name and store it in a safe place until the client is ready to take them.

5. Which of the following reflects acceptable technique when a medication needs to be administered through a gastrostomy tube?
   a. Crushing a Procan SR capsule.
   b. Dissolving a liquid-filled Procardia capsule in warm water.
   c. Crushing an EC-ASA (aspirin) tablet.
   d. Opening an Ornade spansule and dissolving the beads of medication in orange juice.

6. To locate the ventrogluteal site for IM injection, the nurse should:
   a. Divide 1 buttock into quadrants and choose a site in the outer lower quadrant.
   b. Place the palm of the hand over the greater trochanter and point the index finger at the anterior superior iliac spine and the middle finger at the iliac crest.
   c. Place the palm of the hand over the greater trochanter and point the index finger at the iliac crest and the middle finger at the posterior superior iliac spine.
   d. Draw an imaginary line from the posterior superior iliac spine to the greater trochanter and choose a site outside this line.

7. Mr. Rizzo's insulin order reads "15 units Humulin N and 5 units Humulin R." To administer Mr. Rizzo's insulin, the nurse should:
   a. Have the pharmacist prepare a vial of 75% NPH (neutral protamine Hagedorn) and 25% regular Humulin and administer 20 units from this vial.

b. Draw up the ordered amounts of Humulin N and Humulin R in 2 separate syringes.

   c. After injecting air into both vials, draw up the Humulin N, followed by the Humulin R, into the same syringe.

   d. After injecting air into both vials, draw up the Humulin R, followed by the Humulin N, into the same syringe.

8. To administer medication by the sublingual route correctly, the nurse should:

   a. Place the medication in the pocket between the cheek and gum.

   b. Place the medication against the blood vessels visible under the tongue.

   c. Inject the medication at a 10° angle under the top layer of skin on the forearm.

   d. Open the capsule and place the medication on the posterior surface of the tongue.

9. To administer a liquid medication to 4-year-old Shawna, the nurse should:

   a. Use a syringe without a needle to place the medication in Shawna's mouth, while an assistant restrains her.

   b. Disguise the medication in chocolate milk or another sweet beverage.

   c. Offer Shawna a choice between taking the medication from a cup or a spoon.

   d. Have Shawna's mother or father administer the medication.

10. Which of the following would be the best site for an IM injection to a 6-month-old infant?

    a. Vastus lateralis.

    b. Dorsogluteal.

    c. Ventrogluteal.

    d. Deltoid.

11. Maria, who is 7 months pregnant, has fractured her femur. The physician prescribes an analgesic for her. The nurse researches the drug and finds that it is classified in pregnancy category C. What nursing action is indicated?

    a. Instruct Maria to take the analgesic according to the physician's instructions and report any decrease in fetal activity.

    b. Instruct Maria to limit use of the analgesic to occasions when the pain becomes intolerable.

    c. Tell Maria that the safety of the drug for the fetus is unknown and suggest that she consult her obstetrician before taking it.

    d. Remind the physician that Maria is pregnant and ask if a drug in a different pregnancy category can be prescribed.

12. Following successful treatment of congestive heart failure in the hospital, 75-year-old Mr. Tran is to be discharged with prescriptions for digoxin, furosemide, and captopril. To increase the probability that Mr. Tran will comply with his medication regimen, the nurse should:

    a. Tell Mr. Tran to follow the medication schedule established in the hospital.

    b. Plan Mr. Tran's medication schedule to coincide with mealtimes.

    c. Tell Mr. Tran to take the pills at least 1 hour apart.

    d. Assess Mr. Tran's usual routine and help him plan a medication schedule.

ANSWERS

1. **Correct answer is b.** Companies that market generic drugs must demonstrate that their formulations contain the same amount of active drug and achieve the same therapeutic effects before their products may be substituted for brand-name forms.

   a. Physician's permission is not required. If the physician prefers that generic drugs not be substituted, this must be written on the prescription.

   c. Generic drugs do not have to be identical to brand-name drugs as long as they meet the criteria for bioequivalence.

d. When dispensing drugs to outpatients, pharmacists usually ask their preference, but this is not a legal requirement. In hospitals and other health care facilities, substitutions are often made without consulting the client.

2. **Correct answer is c.** Schedule II substances, because they have high abuse potential, are dispensed only by written prescription.

   a. Schedule V drugs, which consist of small amounts of narcotics used as antidiarrheals or antitussives in combination products, can be dispensed over the counter.
   b. Schedule III and IV drugs can be dispensed with a written or oral prescription. Oral prescriptions are permitted because these drugs are considered to have lower abuse potential.
   d. Schedule I drugs, which have no established medical uses, can be dispensed only to participants in approved research studies.

3. **Correct answer is a.** This order includes drug name, dosage, route, and frequency.

   b. The dosage in this order is not sufficiently specific. Units of measure are not specified. The order should say "tabs ii."
   c. Route is not included in this order.
   d. PRN orders must include acceptable frequency of administration, e.g., "every 4 hours."

4. **Correct answer is d.** Since medications may not be returned to the original container after being poured into a medicine cup, the best procedure is to label the cup with client's name and store it in his drawer of the medication cart or another location where it is safe from tampering.

   a. Medications are not to be left at the bedside unless there is a specific order to do so. The nurse should never document medication administration before the client actually takes it.

b. Although having the client inform the nurse when the medication is taken would be more appropriate for correct documentation, it is still inappropriate to leave medications at the bedside.
c. Medications may not be returned to the original container.

5. **Correct answer is b.** Dissolving the liquid-filled capsule in water is the most desirable method, since it assures that the client receives all medication.

   a. SR in the name of a medication indicates that it is a sustained-release form. Crushing a sustained-release capsule would make all medication available for absorption immediately, which might lead to overdose.
   c. EC in the name of the drug indicates it has an enteric coating. Enteric-coated medications should not be crushed, as doing so would eliminate the stomach-protection feature that was the reason for prescribing them.
   d. Spansules are sustained-release forms of medication. They may be opened if the beads are kept intact, but crushing or dissolving the beads would make all medication available at once.

6. **Correct answer is b.** The ventrogluteal site is a wedge of muscle bounded by the anterior superior iliac spine, the iliac crest, and the greater trochanter, which is free of large nerves and blood vessels.

   a. Injection into the outer lower quadrant of the buttock would be an unsafe choice, because there would be a high risk of injection into the sciatic nerve, large blood vessels, or the femoral bone.
   c. This method would result in injection posterior to the correct site.
   d. This describes the dorsogluteal site.

7. **Correct answer is d.** Different types of insulin can be mixed in 1 syringe safely. Regular insulin should be drawn up first. If the intermediate-acting insulin were

inadvertently contaminated with a minute amount of regular insulin, any change in the peak effect of the insulin would occur during the expected duration of action, while monitoring for hypoglycemia would detect it. If obvious contamination of the intermediate-acting insulin occurred, the vial would have to be discarded.

a. A mixture of insulin prepared by the pharmacist would not be stable. Drug companies produce a stable mixture in a 70/30 ratio, but the physician must order its use.
b. Using 2 syringes would be undesirable, due to the discomfort of 2 injections and the increased risk of complications, such as lipodystrophy, if this practice were continued over a long period of time.
c. As noted under correct answer d, regular insulin should be drawn up first. If an undetectable amount of intermediate-acting insulin contaminated the regular insulin vial, the duration of action could be extended beyond that expected, resulting in dangerous adverse reactions.

8. **Correct answer is b.** The word *sublingual* means "under the tongue." For best absorption, the medication should be placed near the capillary beds on the floor of the mouth.

    a. Administration through the pocket between cheek and gum is termed the buccal route.
    c. Injection under the top layer of skin is termed the intradermal route.
    d. Placing medication on the tongue is not an appropriate method for medication administration.

9. **Correct answer is c.** Allowing the preschooler to make some choices will give her a sense of control over the situation, enhancing her compliance.

    a. Using the syringe to place medication in the mouth would be more appropriate for an infant, although the nurse should restrain the infant by holding her close rather than

bringing in another person, which might frighten the infant more.
b. If Shawna fails to drink all of the beverage, the nurse will have no way to know how much of the medication she has actually received. In addition, giving a child the impression that medicine has a sweet taste could contribute to an episode of accidental poisoning.
d. It is undesirable to have the child associate unpleasant procedures with her parents. In addition, if she develops the habit of taking medications only from her parents, the nurse will have increased difficulty with drug administration when the parents are not available.

10. **Correct answer is a.** Because the infant actively moves its arms and legs, the muscles of the thigh (vastus lateralis and rectus femoris) are well developed.

    b and **c.** Because the gluteal muscles are not well developed until the child has been walking for a year, this would be a poor choice.
    d. Although well developed, the deltoid is a poor choice because it is very small in the infant.

11. **Correct answer is d.** Drugs in pregnancy category C should be used only if potential benefits justify the risk to the fetus. Pain management would not justify this risk, since safer analgesics are available.

    a and **b.** Maria should not be told to use the drug until the order is clarified with the physician. Before ordering a drug in this category, the physician should inform Maria of the potential risks to the fetus, so that she can make an informed decision about using the drug.
    c. Maria should inform her obstetrician of any drugs she is taking. However, since category C drugs should not be used when there are safer alternatives, the best initial action is d. Answer c might be appropriate if the

physician refused to change the order even after being informed of Maria's pregnancy and the status of the drug in pregnancy category C.

12. **Correct answer is d.** Deficits in short-term memory are common in Mr. Tran's age group. He is most likely to remember to take his medications if they are scheduled to coincide with significant events in his daily routine. Participating in planning his own medication schedule increases the probability that he will follow it.

a. The hospital schedule is unlikely to fit Mr. Tran's lifestyle. If medication times conflict with his usual activities, he is likely to skip doses.

b. Scheduling medications at mealtimes is one way of helping clients remember to take them. However, Mr. Tran may not eat regular meals, so this may not work for him. If the nurse plans the schedule without his input, his compliance is not promoted.

c. There is no indication that these medications are incompatible, so taking them at different times is not necessary. Limiting the number of times that medication must be taken increases the probability of compliance.

3

Drugs Affecting the Central and Autonomic Nervous Systems

VIII. Anticonvulsants
   A. Hydantoins
   B. Barbiturates
   C. Miscellaneous agents
   D. Nursing diagnoses
   E. Nursing implementation factors
   F. Nursing evaluations

IX. Antiparkinsonian agents
   A. Anticholinergic agents
   B. Dopaminergic agents
   C. Nursing diagnoses
   D. Nursing implementation factors
   E. Nursing evaluations

X. Central nervous system stimulants
   A. Anorexiants
   B. Amphetamines
   C. Other central nervous system stimulants
   D. Methylxanthines
   E. Nursing diagnoses
   F. Nursing implementation factors
   G. Nursing evaluations

XI. Skeletal muscle relaxants
   A. Examples
   B. Use/mechanism of action
   C. Adverse effects
   D. Contraindications
   E. Precautions
   F. Drug interactions
   G. Nursing diagnoses
   H. Nursing implementation factors
   I. Nursing evaluations

NURSING HIGHLIGHTS

1. Analgesics are most effective if administered before pain becomes severe or intolerable.
2. The nurse should focus on relief of pain as it is perceived by the client, not as perceived by the nurse. The nurse must possess accurate, excellent pain assessment skills.
3. Because adrenergic and cholinergic agents affect multiple organ systems, the nurse should give extra time to questioning and monitoring adverse effects in clients receiving these drugs.

GLOSSARY

acetylcholine—a neurotransmitter at cholinergic synapses in the central, sympathetic, and parasympathetic nervous systems

adrenergic agent—a compound that produces responses similar to those obtained when the sympathetic nervous system is activated; also called a sympathomimetic

benzodiazepine—a member of a group of drugs that have antianxiety, hypnotic and sedative, and muscle-relaxing effects

catecholamine—a subtype of adrenergic agents, including endogenous (dopamine, epinephrine, norepinephrine) and synthetic (isoproterenol hydrochloride, dobutamine hydrochloride) agents

cholinergic agent—a drug that directly or indirectly promotes acetylcholine function; also called a parasympathomimetic because it produces responses similar to those produced when the parasympathetic nervous system is stimulated

endorphin—an endogenous polypeptide brain substance that binds to opiate receptors in the brain and thus raises the pain threshold

muscarinic receptor—a type of cholinergic receptor located in the smooth muscle, cardiac muscle, and glands of the parasympathetic fibers and the effector organs of the cholinergic sympathetic fibers

narcotic—a drug that produces insensibility or stupor

opioid—an agent that produces analgesia with loss of consciousness

ENHANCED OUTLINE

I. General anesthetics

See text pages

A. Inhalation anesthetics
1. Examples: enflurane (Ethrane), isoflurane (Forane), nitrous oxide, etomidate, halothane (see Nurse Alert, "Halothane Hepatitis")
2. Use/mechanism of action: cause central nervous system (CNS) depression by producing loss of consciousness, unresponsiveness to pain stimuli, and muscle relaxation
3. Adverse effects: hypotension, prolonged respiratory depression, prolonged recovery, cardiopulmonary depression, confusion, sedation, nausea, vomiting, ataxia, hypothermia
4. Contraindications: hepatic disease, malignant hyperthermia
5. Precautions: pregnancy, lactation
6. Drug interactions
   a) Alcohol: higher dose required to achieve anesthesia
   b) Labetalol, ketamine: hypotension
   c) Other CNS depressants: increased CNS and respiratory depression, hypotension
   d) Xanthines, catecholamines: cardiac arrhythmias
   e) Neuromuscular blocking agents: increased neuromuscular paralysis

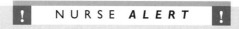

! NURSE *ALERT* !

Halothane Hepatitis

Halothane hepatitis is a very rare but potentially fatal side effect of halothane use. Symptoms are rash, fever, jaundice, nausea, vomiting, eosinophilia, and altered liver functioning.

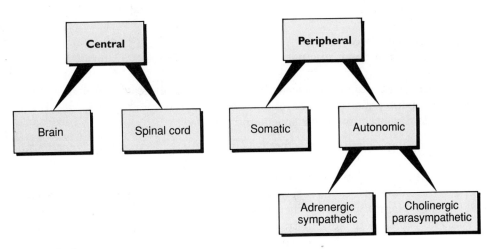

Figure 3–1
Divisions of the Nervous System

      f) Ritodrine: hypotension, cardiac arrhythmias

      g) Succinylcholine: neuromuscular blockade, malignant hypothermia, bradycardia (with repeated use)

      h) Enflurane and isoniazid: nephrotoxicity

      i) Methoxyflurane with aminoglycosides, tetracyclines, or barbiturates: nephrotoxicity

B. Injection anesthetics
    1. Examples: fentanyl (Sublimaze, Innovar [fentanyl and droperidol]); ketamine (Ketalar); thiopental sodium (Pentothal); etomidate (Amidate)
    2. Use/mechanism of action: cause CNS depression by producing loss of consciousness, unresponsiveness to pain stimuli, and muscle relaxation
    3. Adverse effects: hypotension, prolonged respiratory depression, prolonged recovery, cardiopulmonary depression, confusion, sedation, nausea, vomiting, ataxia, hypothermia, muscle rigidity
    4. Contraindications: porphyria
    5. Precautions: cardiovascular disease, pregnancy
    6. Drug interactions
      a) Etomidate
        (1) Antidepressants, CNS-depressant antihypertensives, magnesium sulfate, MAO (monoamine oxidase) inhibitors: increased CNS depression
        (2) Hypotensive agents: increased hypotension
      b) Ketamine
        (1) Inhalation anesthetics: increased hypotension
        (2) CNS-depressant antihypertensives: increased hypotension and respiratory depression

C. Nursing diagnoses
   1. Ineffective breathing pattern related to adverse respiratory effects of anesthetic
   2. Altered thought processes related to prolonged recovery from anesthetic
   3. Hypothermia related to inhalation anesthetic
   4. Pain related to muscle spasm and rigidity

D. Nursing implementation factors (see Nurse Alert, "Malignant Hyperthermic Crisis")
   1. Administration procedures
      a) Monitor client's respiratory status during anesthesia and recovery.
      b) Monitor client's body temperature during and after inhalation anesthetic administration.
      c) Assess client for discomfort due to incomplete anesthesia and after recovery from anesthesia.
      d) Keep resuscitative equipment and emergency drugs at hand.
   2. Daily monitoring and measurements
      a) Monitor client's fluid intake and output.
      b) Monitor client's vital signs before, during, and after anesthesia.
   3. Points for client teaching
      a) Instruct client not to eat or drink for at least 8 hours before anesthesia administration.
      b) Advise client that psychomotor skills may be impaired for 24 hours or more following general anesthesia.
      c) Tell client not to drink alcohol or take any other CNS depressant for 24 hours after anesthesia.

E. Nursing evaluations
   1. Client maintains adequate ventilation during anesthesia.
   2. Client displays normal thought processes after anesthesia.
   3. Client's body temperature returns to normal.
   4. Client shows no signs of pain during anesthesia.

! NURSE *ALERT* !

Malignant Hyperthermic Crisis

Malignant hyperthermic crisis can be triggered in genetically predisposed clients by inhalation anesthetics, depolarizing muscle relaxants, and curare-like neuromuscular blocking agents. Dantrolene is the drug of choice to avoid or treat this potentially fatal response.

II. Analgesics

See text pages
_____

A. Narcotic analgesics
   1. Examples: codeine, meperidine (Demerol), morphine, propoxyphene (Darvon), butorphanol (Stadol), nalbuphine (Nubain), pentazocine (Talwin)
   2. Use/mechanism of action: relieve pain and alter pain perception by binding to opioid receptors in CNS
   3. Adverse effects: respiratory depression, orthostatic hypotension, nausea, vomiting, tolerance, dependence, light-headedness, sedation, euphoria, visual hallucinations, hypertension
   4. Contraindications: MAO inhibitor therapy, known hypersensitivity
   5. Precautions: head injury, increased intracranial or intraocular pressure, hepatic or renal impairment, pregnancy
   6. Drug interactions
      a) Alcohol: CNS and respiratory depression
      b) Barbiturates: additive CNS effects
      c) Cimetidine: inhibition of narcotic metabolism, increasing CNS and respiratory depression
      d) Meperidine and MAO inhibitors: rigidity, hypotension, excitation, increased meperidine effects
      e) Methadone and hydantoins: induction of methadone metabolism, reducing drug effectiveness
      f) Other CNS depressants: increased CNS and respiratory depression

B. Nonnarcotic analgesics
   1. Examples
      a) Nonsteroidal anti-inflammatory drugs (NSAIDs): aspirin (acetylsalicylic acid, ASA); diclofenac sodium (Voltaren); fenoprofen calcium (Nalfon); flurbiprofen (Ansaid); ibuprofen (Motrin); indomethacin (Indocin); ketoprofen (Orudis); ketorolac (Toradol); meclofenamate sodium (Meclomen); naproxen (Naprosyn); piroxicam (Feldene); sulindac (Clinoril); tolmetin sodium (Tolectin)
      b) Other nonnarcotic analgesics: acetaminophen (Tylenol), phenazopyridine hydrochloride (Pyridium)
   2. Use/mechanism of action
      a) Relieve pain and alter pain perception by acting in the peripheral nervous system to inhibit the formation or reactivity of prostaglandins
      b) Reduce inflammatory response triggered by trauma, microorganisms, drugs, or other foreign substances (NSAIDs)
      c) Control fever, probably by inhibiting prostaglandin release (NSAIDs)
   3. Adverse effects
      a) All agents: gastrointestinal (GI) distress and irritation, gastric ulcer, prolonged bleeding time, bruising, dizziness, headache, drowsiness, tinnitus, visual disturbances, edema, abnormal liver function tests
      b) Aspirin: salicylism (adverse effects common to all agents and reversible hearing loss, rash, confusion, nausea, vomiting)

    c) Ibuprofen: nephrotic syndrome, cystitis, dysuria, hematuria, hypoglycemia, hyperglycemia

    d) Indomethacin: fatigue, muscle weakness, ataxia, aggravation of depression or other psychiatric disorders, epilepsy, hyperkalemia, hyperglycemia in diabetics, decreased hemoglobin and hematocrit; reactivation of latent infections

    e) Meclofenamate: agranulocytosis and aplastic anemia, palpitations

    f) Sulindac: dry mouth, decreased hearing, hematologic changes, aplastic anemia

4. Contraindications

    a) All agents: GI bleeding, gastric ulcer, currently active GI disease

    b) Aspirin: flulike illness or chicken pox in children under 18, pregnancy

    c) Ibuprofen: acute asthma, nasal polyps

    d) Indomethacin: lactation, nasal polyps associated with angioedema

    e) Meclofenamate: severe rheumatoid arthritis, severe renal or hepatic impairment

5. Precautions

    a) All agents: hepatic or renal impairment, bleeding or coagulation disorders

    b) Aspirin: hypoprothrombinemia, vitamin K deficiency, aspirin triad (rhinitis, asthma, nasal polyps)

    c) Ibuprofen: advanced age, childhood (birth to age 14), pregnancy

    d) Indomethacin: history of psychiatric disorders, epilepsy, Parkinson's disease, compromised cardiac function, advanced age, childhood, pregnancy

    e) Meclofenamate: impaired cardiovascular function

    f) Sulindac: pregnancy, childhood, advanced age, hypertension, impaired cardiac function

6. Drug interactions

    a) Alcohol: increased ulcerogenic effect of salicylates; increased risk of hepatoxicity when used on long-term basis in conjunction with acetaminophen

    b) Oral anticoagulants and heparin: increased anticoagulant effect and risk of bleeding with salicylates

    c) Corticosteroids: decreased plasma salicylate concentrations and increased ulcerogenic effect of salicylates

    d) Methotrexate: increased effect and toxicity of methotrexate when taken with salicylates

    e) Cholestyramine, colestipol: reduced GI absorption of acetaminophen

    f) Antihypertensives, diuretics: reduction of antihypertensive effects by NSAIDs

g) Probenecid: increased NSAID serum level, heightening risk of toxicity

h) Antacids: decreased effects of NSAIDs

C. Nursing diagnoses
1. Pain related to underlying condition
2. Altered thought processes related to use of narcotic analgesic
3. High risk for injury related to GI side effects and prolonged bleeding time of nonnarcotic analgesic
4. Sensory, perceptual alteration related to use of narcotic analgesic
5. Anxiety related to unrelieved pain
6. Potential respiratory depression related to use of narcotic analgesic
7. Impaired mobility related to inflammatory disorder

D. Nursing implementation factors
1. Administration procedures
   a) Monitor respiratory status during and after administration.
   b) Have respiratory support equipment at hand.
   c) Do not discontinue narcotics abruptly in the narcotic-dependent client.
   d) Do not mix pentazocine with a barbiturate in the same syringe.
2. Daily monitoring and measurements
   a) Determine level of pain and effectiveness of analgesics.
   b) Monitor vital signs.
   c) Measure respiratory rate, pattern, and depth.
   d) Watch for signs of dependence.
   e) Encourage clients to achieve optimal pain control by taking medication before pain becomes severe.
   f) Teach client nonpharmacologic pain relief measures to augment analgesic use.
   g) Measure white blood cell count (WBC) at regular intervals in patients receiving nonnarcotic agents.
   h) Monitor hemoglobin and/or hematocrit in patients receiving nonnarcotic agents.
3. Points for client teaching
   a) Caution client that alertness may be impaired.
   b) Tell client to avoid concomitant use of alcohol and other CNS depressants.
   c) Tell client not to give drug to friends or family members.
   d) Warn client about possibility of dependence.
   e) Caution female client of childbearing age that NSAIDs may interfere with blood clotting and prolong duration of pregnancy and labor.
   f) Teach client to take NSAID with a full glass of water and to remain in an upright position for 30 minutes.
   g) Advise client to take NSAID with meals to decrease the risk of gastrointestinal side effects.

E. Nursing evaluations
1. Client reports relief of pain.
2. Client maintains normal mental functioning and mood.

3. Client avoids GI injury.
4. Client is able to perform necessary activities (e.g., coughing and turning).
5. Client's anxiety is relieved as pain control is achieved.
6. Client taking NSAID shows reduced signs of inflammation, including pain, swelling, and redness.
7. Client taking NSAID experiences improved comfort, range of motion, and ability to perform activities of daily living.
8. Client takes NSAID with food to avoid gastric upset.

See text pages

_____

III. Cholinergic agents (parasympathomimetics)

A. Examples: synthetic acetylcholine; bethanechol (Duvoid, Myotonachol, Urecholine); carbachol (Carbacel, Isopto Carbachol, Miostat); pilocarpine (Adsorbocarpine, Akarpine, Isopto Carpine, Pilocar); ambenonium (Mytelase); edrophonium (Tensilon); neostigmine (Prostigmin); pyridostigmine bromide (Mestinon)

B. Use/mechanism of action: treat glaucoma, urine retention, and myasthenia gravis; serve as an antidote to neuromuscular blocking agents, tricyclic antidepressants, and belladonna alkaloids through stimulation of cholinergic receptors by mimicking acetylcholine or inhibition of enzyme acetylcholinesterase to prolong action of acetylcholine

C. Adverse effects
   1. Eye: blurred vision, decreased accommodation, miosis
   2. Skin: diaphoresis
   3. GI: increased salivation, belching, nausea, vomiting, intestinal cramps, diarrhea
   4. Respiratory: bronchoconstriction, including shortness of breath, tightness in chest, wheezing
   5. Cardiovascular: vasodilation and hypotension, bradycardia
   6. CNS: irritability, anxiety, seizures

D. Contraindications: GI or urinary obstruction, peritonitis

E. Precautions: ulcers, GI inflammation, pregnancy, coronary disease, hyperthyroidism, asthma, cardiac arrhythmias, epilepsy

F. Drug interactions
   1. Anticholinesterase agents and cholinergic agonists: intensification of each other's effects, increasing risk of toxicity
   2. Cholinergic blocking agents (e.g., atropine): antagonism of acetylcholine's effect at muscarinic receptors, serving as antidote
   3. Ester anesthetics: increased risk of toxicity from anticholinesterase agents

4. Ganglionic blocking agents: severe GI distress and hypotension
5. Procainamide and quinidine: antagonism of cholinergics

G. Nursing diagnoses
  1. Altered urinary elimination related to urinary frequency caused by cholinergic agonist
  2. Potential for injury related to adverse GI tract effects

H. Nursing implementation factors (see Nurse Alert, "Heatstroke and Cholinergic Blocking Agents")
  1. Administration procedures
    a) Keep respiratory support equipment nearby.
    b) Have atropine available for use as an antagonist.
    c) Monitor vital signs and auscultate breathing while administering the cholinergic agent.
  2. Daily monitoring and measurements
    a) Check client's vision frequently if an ocular condition is being treated with a cholinergic agent, realizing that visual acuity may be diminished.
    b) Monitor pulse and blood pressure daily.
    c) Report signs of excessive cholinergic activity.
  3. Points for client teaching
    a) Show client how to instill cholinergic agent into eye.
    b) Tell client that drug may affect visual acuity.
    c) Show client receiving anticholinesterase therapy how to assess and record changes in muscle strength.
    d) Help client on anticholinesterase therapy to develop a system for recording each dose and its effect.
    e) Stress need to take drugs on time.

I. Nursing evaluations
  1. Client maintains normal urinary elimination pattern.
  2. Client avoids injury to GI tract.

IV. Cholinergic blocking agents (parasympatholytics, anticholinergics)

See text pages
_____

A. Examples: atropine; belladonna; scopolamine (Transderm Scop, Triptone); dicyclomine (Antispas, Bentyl, Viscerol); propantheline (Pro-Banthine)

B. Use/mechanism of action: treat spasticity of GI or urinary tract, bradycardia, motion sickness, parkinsonism, and chronic asthma by blocking binding of acetylcholine at muscarinic receptors of parasympathetic nerves; also used preoperatively to dry up secretions

C. Adverse effects
1. Decreases in salivation, bronchial secretions, and sweating; increased risk of heatstroke
2. Dilatation of pupils with reduction in accommodation
3. Increased heart rate; atrial and ventricular arrhythmias
4. Urinary retention
5. Decreased intestinal and gastric motility
6. CNS toxicity manifested by restlessness followed by depression, irritability, disorientation, delirium
7. Signs of toxicity that can be remembered as "hot as a hare, blind as a bat, dry as a bone, mad as a hatter"

D. Contraindications: glaucoma, coronary artery disease, renal or GI obstructive disease, reflux esophagitis, myasthenia gravis

E. Precautions: benign prostate enlargement or cardiovascular disease in elderly, coronary heart disease, hypertension, hyperthyroidism, ulcerative colitis, hiatal hernia

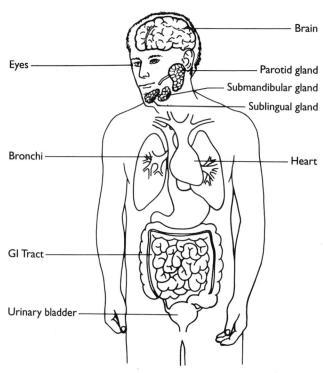

Figure 3–2
Parts of the Body Affected by Cholinergic Blockers

F. Drug interactions
   1. Antidepressants, antidyskinetics, antiemetics, antivertigo drugs, antipsychotics: increased anticholinergic effects
   2. Cholinergic agonists, anticholinesterase drugs: drug antagonism
   3. Digoxin: increased serum concentration
   4. Opioid analgesics: decreased GI motility
   5. Nitroglycerin: delayed sublingual absorption of nitroglycerin

G. Nursing diagnoses
   1. Potential for injury related to risk of heatstroke
   2. Urinary retention related to cholinergic blockers in client with benign prostate enlargement
   3. Constipation related to decreased intestinal motility
   4. Altered oral mucous membranes related to decreased secretions

H. Nursing implementation factors
   1. Administration procedures
      a) If prescribed for GI spasticity, administer 30 minutes before meals and at bedtime.
      b) Keep client's room cool.
   2. Daily monitoring and measurements
      a) Monitor vital signs, including temperature, every 4 hours.
      b) Watch for signs of heatstroke and dehydration.
      c) Measure fluid intake and output, particularly in clients with benign prostate enlargement.
   3. Points for client teaching
      a) Teach client precautions to prevent heatstroke.
      b) Warn client about dangers of toxicity and caution him/her to take only the prescribed dose.
      c) Encourage increased fluid intake and/or use of sugarless gums and candies.
      d) Advise client to avoid late night snacks and milk, which increase gastric secretions.

I. Nursing evaluations
   1. Client avoids dry mouth.
   2. Client maintains normal body temperature.
   3. Client maintains normal urinary frequency and output.
   4. Client shows no signs of GI spasticity, such as abdominal cramps or diarrhea.
   5. Client reports absence of nausea.
   6. Client reports decreased wheezing.
   7. Client's enlarged pupils return to normal size.

V. Adrenergic agents (sympathomimetics)

See text pages
_____

A. Examples
   1. Direct-acting agents
      a) Endogenous catecholamines: epinephrine, norepinephrine, dopamine (Intropin)

   b) Synthetic catecholamines: isoproterenol, dobutamine (Dobutrex)
   c) Other: albuterol, isoetharine, terbutaline
2. Dual-acting agents: ephedrine (Ephed II), phenylephrine (Neo-Synephrine), mephentermine, metaraminol (Aramine), methoxamine (Vasoxyl)
3. Agents classified by receptor affected
   a) $Beta_1$ activity: dobutamine, norepinephrine, epinephrine, isoproterenol
   b) $Beta_2$ activity: epinephrine, ritodrine, terbutaline, isoproterenol, albuterol, isoetharine
   c) Alpha activity: epinephrine, methoxamine, metaraminol, phenylephrine, norepinephrine

B. Use/mechanism of action
   1. Purposes
      a) To treat hypotension (norepinephrine and alpha-agonists)
      b) To treat bradycardia, heart block occurring with Stokes-Adams syndrome and carotid sinus syndrome, insufficient cardiac output ($beta_1$-agonists)
      c) To treat asthma, emphysema, bronchitis, and acute drug hypersensitivity ($beta_2$-agonists)
      d) To treat allergic reactions, anaphylactic shock, acute hypotension, shock, and cardiac arrest (epinephrine)
      e) To treat nasal and ophthalmic congestion (catecholamines, because of their vasoconstrictive effects)
   2. Use/mechanism of action
      a) Catecholamines and other direct-acting adrenergics: stimulate alpha- and beta-adrenergic receptors directly
         (1) Norepinephrine and alpha-agonists: act mainly on alpha-receptors, causing vasoconstriction of arterioles in skin, kidneys, mesentery, and splanchnic area; raising blood pressure; dilating the pupils; and relaxing the gut
         (2) Beta-agonists: cause vasodilation of arterioles supplying brain, heart, and skeletal muscle; induce cardiac stimulation, bronchial and uterine (smooth muscle) relaxation
         (3) Epinephrine: acts on both alpha- and beta-receptors, causing a combined response of vasoconstriction and vasodilation
         (4) Dopamine and dopaminergic agonists: act on dopamine receptors in CNS; also act indirectly, stimulating norepinephrine release
      b) Indirect-acting adrenergics: trigger release of a catecholamine, usually norepinephrine
      c) Dual-acting adrenergics: combine direct and indirect action

C. Adverse effects (differing from drug to drug)
   1. CNS: restlessness, anxiety, dizziness, headache, insomnia
   2. Cardiovascular: palpitations, cardiac arrhythmias, tachycardia, hypertension, cerebrovascular accidents, angina
   3. Skeletal muscle: weakness, tremors
   4. GI: nausea, severe vomiting, diarrhea
   5. Skin: local necrosis and tissue sloughing from extravasated intravenous (IV) catecholamines

D. Contraindications: cardiovascular disease, pheochromocytoma, hypertension

E. Precautions: hyperthyroidism, diabetes, pregnancy

F. Drug interactions
   1. Alpha-blockers (e.g., phentolamine): antagonism of alpha-agonists, resulting in hypotension
   2. Beta-blockers and alpha-agonists: mutually antagonistic, possibly allowing alpha effects to predominate, resulting in hypertension
   3. Oral hypoglycemic agents: hyperglycemia
   4. Adrenergic agents used together: additive effect, producing hypertension, cardiac arrhythmias, and increased adverse effects
   5. Blood products and heparin: incompatible with adrenergic agents

G. Nursing diagnoses
   1. Urinary retention related to stimulation of alpha-and beta-adrenergic receptors
   2. Anxiety related to CNS effects
   3. Potential for injury related to dizziness and vertigo

H. Nursing implementation factors
   1. Administration procedures: Administer dopamine hydrochloride only by intravenous infusion, using a dedicated line.
   2. Daily monitoring and measurements
      a) Measure glucose levels in client with diabetes.
      b) Monitor electrocardiogram, blood pressure, cardiac rate, and cardiac rhythm during infusion.
   3. Points for client teaching
      a) Teach client how to measure pulse rate and when to report it.
      b) Show client how to use inhalant device.
      c) Advise client to use smallest number of inhalations to accomplish drug administration and to minimize dry mouth by rinsing mouth after inhalation.
      d) Caution client with diabetes to notify physician of changes in glucose test results or symptoms of hyperglycemia.

I. Nursing evaluations (dependent on desired effect and use of drug)
   1. Client is able to perform usual activities without impairment.
   2. Client maintains normal mental functioning and mood.
   3. Client avoids dehydration.
   4. Client avoids CNS adverse effects.
   5. Client has no tissue damage from catecholamine extravasation.

See text pages
_____

VI. Adrenergic blocking agents (sympatholytics)

A. Alpha-blockers

1. Examples: phenoxybenzamine (Dibenzyline), phentolamine (Regitine), ergotamine tartrate (Ergomar)

2. Use/mechanism of action: treat Raynaud's disease, hypertension secondary to pheochromocytoma, and migraine (ergotamine) by inhibiting action of alpha-receptors in vascular smooth muscle, causing vasodilation

3. Adverse effects (see Nurse Alert, "Ergotamine Toxicity")

   a) Cardiovascular: orthostatic hypotension or severe hypertensive episodes, bradycardia or tachycardia, edema, dyspnea, angina, myocardial infarction, cerebrovascular spasm

   b) CNS: paresthesias, muscle weakness, fatigue, depression, insomnia, lethargy, sedation, vertigo, syncope, confusion, headache

   c) Ear, nose, throat: nasal congestion, tinnitus, dry mouth

   d) GI: nausea, vomiting, heartburn, diarrhea, cramping, exacerbated peptic ulcers

   e) Genitourinary: urinary frequency, incontinence, impotence, priapism

4. Contraindications: myocardial infarction, coronary insufficiency, angina

5. Precautions: pregnancy, lactation

6. Drug interactions

   a) Ergotamine and nitroglycerine: excessive vasodilation and increased ergot availability

   b) Other hypertensives: potentiation of hypotensive effects

B. Beta-blockers

1. Examples

   a) Selective beta-blockers: acebutolol (Sectral), atenolol (Tenormin), esmolol hydrochloride (Brevibloc), metoprolol tartrate (Lopressor)

   b) Nonselective beta-blockers: carteolol hydrochloride (Cartrol), labetalol hydrochloride (Normodyne), nadolol (Corgard), penbutolol sulfate (Levatol), propranolol (Inderal), timolol (Blocadren)

2. Use/mechanism of action: treat hypertension, angina, arrhythmias, migraine, idiopathic hypertrophic subaortic stenosis, mitral valve prolapse, glaucoma, and other disorders by competing with epinephrine

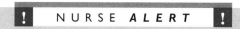

! NURSE **ALERT** !

Ergotamine Toxicity

Ergotism from ergotamine toxicity results in prolonged vasoconstriction marked by cold, numb extremities; diminished or absent arterial peripheral pulse; seizures; and tissue damage, including gangrene.

to occupy beta-adrenergic receptors in heart (beta$_1$) and/or peripheral circulation, pulmonary airways, and CNS (beta$_2$)

3. Adverse effects
    a) Cardiovascular: arrhythmias, orthostatic hypotension, bradycardia, congestive heart failure, edema, cold extremities
    b) CNS: fatigue, vivid dreams, depression, insomnia, vertigo
    c) GI: nausea, vomiting, diarrhea, constipation
    d) Respiratory: bronchospasm, dyspnea
    e) Skin: rash, pruritus
    f) Hematologic: hyperglycemia, hypoglycemia
4. Contraindications: congestive heart failure, sinus bradycardia, heart block, cardiogenic shock, bronchospastic disease
5. Precautions: diabetes, hypoglycemia, hepatic or renal impairment, respiratory disease
6. Drug interactions
    a) Antacids: delayed absorption from GI tract
    b) Lidocaine: increased plasma levels of lidocaine and increased risk of potential toxicity
    c) Insulin and oral hypoglycemic agents: hypoglycemia or hyperglycemia
    d) Anti-inflammatory agents: decreased hypotensive effects of beta-blockers
    e) Barbiturates: stimulation of beta-blocker metabolism in liver
    f) Cimetidine: metabolism reduced
    g) Cardiac glycosides: additive bradycardia and depressed atrioventricular conduction
    h) Calcium channel blockers: mutually increased therapeutic and adverse effects
    i) Sympathomimetics: hypertension and reflex bradycardia
    j) Theophyllines: impaired bronchodilation
    k) Clonidine: severe hypertension
    l) Halothane anesthetics: increased hypotension

C. Nursing diagnoses
    1. Potential for injury related to adverse CNS effects
    2. Activity intolerance related to adverse CNS effects
    3. Ineffective breathing pattern related to respiratory depression
    4. Fatigue related to adverse CNS effects

D. Nursing implementation factors
    1. Administration procedures
        a) Alpha-blockers
            (1) Administer oral drugs with milk to minimize GI effects.
            (2) Administer ergotamine early in a migraine attack, while reducing light and noise in client's environment.
        b) Beta-blockers
            (1) Administer oral drug before meals or at bedtime to speed absorption.
            (2) Refrain from administering in evening if insomnia occurs.

IV. Cholinergic blocking agents	V. Adrenergic agents	VI. Adrenergic blocking agents	VII. Neuromuscular blocking agents	VIII. Anticonvulsants

          (3) Administer any needed antacids several hours before or after beta-blocker administration.

          (4) Check client's apical pulse rate before drug administration; if under 60, inform physician before proceeding.

    2. Daily monitoring and measurements

      a) Alpha-blockers

        (1) Note any change in blood pressure when client rises from supine position.

        (2) Auscultate breath sounds.

        (3) Note signs and symptoms of light-headedness, weakness, or altered mental functioning. Elevate client's bed side rails and give assistance if CNS symptoms occur.

        (4) Monitor client taking ergotamine for signs of vascular insufficiency, including numbness, coldness, tingling, or weakness in extremities.

        (5) Notify physician immediately if client reports chest pain.

      b) Beta-blockers

        (1) Monitor vital signs, fluid intake and output, breath sounds, and peripheral circulation before and during drug administration.

        (2) Monitor blood glucose levels in clients with diabetes.

        (3) Use safety precautions, including use of bed side rails, if client develops adverse CNS effects.

    3. Points for client teaching

      a) Advise client to avoid drinking alcohol when taking an alpha-blocker.

      b) Tell client to avoid over-the-counter (OTC) medications that contain alcohol or caffeine unless physician has approved them.

      c) Show client methods for minimizing the effects of orthostatic hypotension, dizziness, and light-headedness.

      d) Warn client not to drive or operate dangerous machinery until he/she has adjusted to medication.

      e) Encourage client to monitor weight.

      f) Teach client to monitor pulse and blood pressure.

  E. Nursing evaluations

    1. Client's blood pressure is within normal range.

    2. Client's arrhythmia is controlled.

    3. Client reports decrease or absence of chest pain.

    4. Client can demonstrate proper management of orthostatic hypotension.

    5. Client reports relief of migraine headache.

    6. Client can correctly measure pulse rate.

    7. Client has adequate cardiopulmonary tissue perfusion.

    8. Client maintains adequate nutrition and body weight.

VII. Neuromuscular blocking agents

See text pages
_____

A. Nondepolarizing agents
   1. Examples: atracurium (Tracrium), pancuronium (Pavulon), pipecuronium (Arduan), tubocurarine (Tubarine), vecuronium (Norcuron)
   2. Use/mechanism of action: relax skeletal muscle during surgery, minimize muscle spasms during electroconvulsive therapy, and relax clients during intubation or mechanical ventilation by blocking acetylcholine at cholinergic receptors in skeletal muscle membrane, preventing depolarization and contraction
   3. Adverse effects: hypotension and bronchospasm; increased bronchial and salivary secretions
   4. Contraindications: bromide hypersensitivity
   5. Precautions: renal, hepatic, cardiac, or pulmonary impairment; fluid and electrolyte imbalance; myasthenia gravis
   6. Drug interactions
      a) Inhalation anesthetics, aminoglycosides, clindamycin, polymyxin, calcium channel blockers, magnesium salts, potassium-depleting agents: potentiation of effects of nondepolarizing agents
      b) Anticholinesterase agents: antagonism of nondepolarizing agents

B. Succinylcholine
   1. Example: succinylcholine (Anectine)
   2. Use/mechanism of action: relax skeletal muscle during surgery, minimize muscle spasms during electroconvulsive therapy, and relax clients during intubation or mechanical ventilation by mimicking acetylcholine to depolarize postsynaptic muscle membrane, resulting in repeated contractions followed by muscle paralysis
   3. Adverse effects: apnea, hypotension, and bronchospasm; increased bronchial and salivary secretions, muscle pain
   4. Contraindications: malignant hyperthermia, acute narrow-angle glaucoma, penetrating eye injury, myopathy
   5. Precautions: renal, pulmonary, or neuromuscular disorder; fluid and electrolyte imbalance; increased intraocular pressure; family history of malignant hyperthermia
   6. Drug interactions
      a) Anesthetics and antibiotics (some): potentiation of succinylcholine
      b) Anticholinesterase agents: intensification of neuromuscular blockade

C. Nursing diagnoses
   1. Potential for injury related to CNS effects
   2. Anxiety related to muscle paralysis
   3. Impaired communication related to muscle paralysis
   4. Ineffective breathing pattern related to respiratory muscle paralysis

D. Nursing implementation factors
   1. Administration procedures
      a) Keep antagonists at hand.
      b) Have endotracheal equipment, suction equipment, oxygen, and mechanical ventilator available for emergency.

         c) Administer these agents in conjunction with an anxiolytic.

         d) Monitor vital signs and respiratory rate and pattern during succinylcholine infusion.

     2. Daily monitoring and measurements

         a) Monitor respirations until client recovers completely from neuromuscular blockade.

         b) Suction client as necessary.

         c) Monitor serum potassium level during succinylcholine infusion.

         d) Monitor intake and output of fluids and electrolyte levels in client with renal disease receiving nondepolarizing agent.

     3. Points for client teaching

         a) Inform client beforehand of all procedures to minimize anxiety.

         b) Encourage client to ask questions to alleviate anxiety.

  E. Nursing evaluations

     1. Client maintains adequate ventilation during neuromuscular blockade.

     2. Client is relaxed and free from anxiety during neuromuscular blockade.

VIII. Anticonvulsants

See text pages

A. Hydantoins

     1. Examples: phenytoin (Dilantin), mephenytoin (Mesantoin), ethotoin (Peganone)

     2. Use/mechanism of action: treat seizures by depressing abnormal neuronal activity in motor cortex to prevent spread of seizure activity

     3. Adverse effects: drowsiness, gingival hyperplasia, blood dyscrasias, nausea, vomiting, anorexia, hypersensitivity reactions

     4. Contraindications: hypoglycemia-induced seizures, sinus bradycardia, heart block, Adams-Stokes syndrome

     5. Precautions: childhood, advanced age, pregnancy, lactation, impaired liver or kidney function, alcoholism, hypotension, myocardial insufficiency, heart failure, pancreatic adenoma, diabetes mellitus, hyperglycemia, respiratory depression

     6. Drug interactions

         a) Cimetidine, disulfiram, isoniazid, sulfonamides, chloramphenicol, amiodarone: inhibition of phenytoin metabolism, increasing risk of toxicity

         b) Corticosteroids, doxycycline, methadone, metyrapone, quinidine, mexiletine, thyroid hormone, oral contraceptives: induction of metabolism of these drugs, decreasing their efficacy

B. Barbiturates

     1. Examples: phenobarbital (Luminal), mephobarbital (Mebaral), primidone (Mysoline)

2. Use/mechanism of action: treat seizures by depressing abnormal neuronal activity in motor cortex to prevent spread of seizure activity
3. Adverse effects: dizziness, drowsiness, nausea, vomiting, hypotension, respiratory depression
4. Contraindications: porphyria
5. Precautions: renal or hepatic disease, diabetes, borderline hypoadrenal function, history of drug abuse
6. Drug interactions
   a) Alcohol, antihistamines, narcotics, benzodiazepines, MAO (monoamine oxidase) inhibitors, methylphenidate, isoniazid, CNS depressants: excessive sedation
   b) Griseofulvin: decreased griseofulvin absorption
   c) Oral anticoagulants: increased metabolism of oral anticoagulants

C. Miscellaneous agents
1. Examples: carbamazepine (Tegretol), diazepam (Valium), clorazepate (Tranxene), clonazepam (Klonopin), ethosuximide (Zarontin), methsuximide (Celontin), phensuximide (Milontin), valproic acid (Depakene, Depakote)
2. Use/mechanism of action: treat seizures by depressing abnormal neuronal activity in motor cortex to prevent spread of seizure activity
3. Adverse effects: headache, drowsiness, sedation, confusion, diplopia, nystagmus, vertigo, dizziness, ataxia, tremor, muscle weakness, dry mouth, nausea, vomiting, diarrhea, constipation, thrombocytopenia, agranulocytosis, aplastic anemia, urinary frequency; hepatotoxicity (rare, with valproic acid)
4. Contraindications: history of bone marrow depression
5. Precautions: liver, kidney, cardiovascular disease, pregnancy, lactation
6. Drug interactions
   a) Erythromycin, isoniazid, propoxyphene, troleandomycin, cimetidine: inhibition of iminostilbene metabolism, increasing risk of toxicity
   b) Lithium: induction of neurotoxicity when administered with iminostilbenes
   c) Doxycycline, theophylline, warfarin, oral contraceptives: increased metabolism of these drugs, decreasing their efficacy, with iminostilbene administration
   d) Hydantoin: inhibition of succinimide metabolism
   e) Carbamazepine: decreased concentration of succinimide, reducing its efficacy
   f) Valproic acid and phenobarbital: inhibition of phenobarbital metabolism, increasing risk of toxicity

D. Nursing diagnoses
1. Activity intolerance related to muscle weakness
2. Altered oral mucous membrane related to gum hypertrophy (phenytoin)
3. Potential for injury related to adverse CNS effects

E. Nursing implementation factors
   1. Administration procedures
      a) Administer intravenous (IV) phenytoin slowly (50 mg/minute) to avoid cardiotoxicity.
      b) Monitor blood pressure, pulse, and respiration during phenytoin administration and afterward until client is stable.
      c) Reduce phenytoin infusion rate if blood pressure drops.
      d) Avoid mixing other drugs in same syringe with phenytoin.
      e) Administer barbiturates and benzodiazepines according to the procedures given in section I,E,1 of Chapter 4.
      f) Administer succinimides or valproic acid with food to avoid adverse GI effects.
      g) Avoid intramuscular (IM) or intravenous (IV) administration of valproic acid to reduce chance of bleeding.
   2. Daily monitoring and measurements
      a) Monitor seizure activity.
      b) Monitor serum drug concentration.
      c) Periodically check liver and kidney function tests and blood count.
      d) Monitor client taking phenytoin for signs of hyperglycemia.
      e) Assess client on carbamazepine daily for dependent edema.
      f) Weigh client on carbamazepine daily.
      g) Limit fluid and salt intake of client on carbamazetpine.
      h) Monitor client on succinimides for nutritional deficiencies and encourage a well-balanced diet.
      i) Monitor client's mental status and take precautions if mental status alters.
   3. Points for client teaching
      a) Advise female clients to use contraceptive.
      b) Tell client taking phenytoin or phensuximide that drug may cause harmless urine discoloration.
      c) Warn client with diabetes that hydantoins may increase blood glucose levels and that valproic acid may produce a false-positive result on a urine ketone test.
      d) Teach client receiving carbamazepine to identify early symptoms of hematologic abnormalities, such as fever, sore throat, malaise, unusual fatigue, bleeding, and bruising.
      e) Caution client to take benzodiazepines exactly as prescribed to prevent drug dependence.
      f) Reassure client that barbiturates are not addictive at the low dosage used for seizure control.
F. Nursing evaluations
   1. Client has no seizures.
   2. Client is alert and active.

IX. Antiparkinsonian agents

See text pages

A. Anticholinergic agents
   1. Examples: trihexyphenidyl (Artane, Hexaphen, Trihexane); benztropine (Cogentin); diphenhydramine (Benadryl)
   2. Use/mechanism of action: treat Parkinson's disease and parkinsonism by inhibiting cerebral motor centers
   3. Adverse effects: same as section IV,C of this chapter
   4. Contraindications: same as section IV,D of this chapter
   5. Precautions: same as section IV,E of this chapter
   6. Drug interactions: same as section IV,F of this chapter

B. Dopaminergic agents
   1. Examples: levodopa (Dopar, Larodopa, Levopa); carbidopa-levodopa (Sinemet); pergolide (Permax); amantadine (Symmetrel); selegiline (Eldepryl)
   2. Use/mechanism of action: treat Parkinson's disease and parkinsonism by increasing dopamine concentrations or enhancing neurotransmitter functioning
   3. Adverse effects
      a) Levodopa
         (1) GI: nausea, vomiting, anorexia
         (2) Cardiovascular: orthostatic hypotension, palpitations, tachycardia
         (3) CNS: irritability, confusion, hallucinations
         (4) Other: dark-colored urine and sweat, urinary frequency or retention
      b) Amantadine: livedo reticularis, ankle edema, urine retention, orthostatic hypotension, anorexia, nausea, constipation (all from long-term use)
      c) Bromocriptine
         (1) GI: nausea, vomiting
         (2) Cardiovascular: orthostatic hypotension, ankle edema, palpitations, tachycardia or bradycardia
         (3) CNS: confusion, hallucinations, nightmares
      d) Selegiline: nausea, dry mouth, dizziness, confusion
   4. Contraindications: glaucoma
   5. Precautions: cardiopulmonary, renal, hepatic, or endocrine disease, seizures, psychosis
   6. Drug interactions
      a) Levodopa
         (1) Antipsychotics, anticholinergics, reserpine, benzodiazepines, pyridoxine, phenytoin, papaverine: decreased dopaminergic effects of levodopa
         (2) MAO inhibitors: induction of hypertensive crisis
      b) Pergolide: decreased dopaminergic effects with antipsychotics, reserpine
      c) Amantadine and anticholinergics: increased anticholinergic effects
      d) Selegiline and meperidine: potentially fatal reaction

C. Nursing diagnoses
   1. Potential for injury related to adverse CNS effects
   2. Altered urinary elimination related to adverse effects of antiparkinsonian agent
   3. Impaired mobility related to ineffectiveness of antiparkinsonian agent
   4. Constipation related to adverse GI effects

D. Nursing implementation factors
   1. Administration procedures
      a) Anticholinergic agents: same as section IV,H,1 of this chapter
      b) Dopaminergic agents
         (1) Give after meals to reduce GI symptoms.
         (2) Refrain from administering amantadine late at night if insomnia occurs.
   2. Daily monitoring and measurements
      a) Anticholinergic agents: same as section IV,H,2 of this chapter
      b) Assess client's mobility.
      c) Monitor client's blood pressure.
      d) Elevate client's legs to reduce edema.
   3. Points for client teaching
      a) Warn client not to exceed daily dosage.
      b) Reassure client that levodopa may cause harmless darkening of urine and sweat.
      c) Show client methods of minimizing orthostatic hypotension.
      d) Because scheduling of medications is very client specific, encourage close follow-up.

E. Nursing evaluations
   1. Client achieves good therapeutic effects with antiparkinsonian agent, improving mobility and functioning and decreasing tremors and rigidity.
   2. Client maintains normal mental functioning.
   3. Client maintains normal urinary elimination pattern.

X. Central nervous system stimulants

See text pages

A. Anorexiants
   1. Examples: phentermine (Phentrol), fenfluramine (Pondimin)
   2. Use/mechanism of action: treat obesity by increasing excitatory CNS neurotransmitter activity, blocking inhibitory impulses or otherwise altering neurotransmitter availability and neuronal response
   3. Adverse effects: insomnia, euphoria, nervousness, irritability, dry mouth, restlessness, dependence, tolerance; chorea (with long-term use)
   4. Contraindications: agitation, alcoholism, drug abuse, psychosis, depression; arteriosclerosis, cardiovascular disease, glaucoma, hypertension, uremia, hyperthyroidism

5. Precautions: advanced age or debilitation
6. Drug interactions: hypertensive crisis with MAO inhibitors

B. Amphetamines
1. Examples: amphetamine, dextroamphetamine (Dexedrine), methamphetamine (Desoxyn, Methapex)
2. Use/mechanism of action: treat obesity, attention deficit disorder with hyperactivity, and narcolepsy by increasing excitatory CNS neurotransmitter activity, blocking inhibitory impulses or otherwise altering neurotransmitter availability and neuronal response
3. Adverse effects: insomnia, euphoria, nervousness, irritability, dry mouth, restlessness, dependence, tolerance; chorea (with long-term use)
4. Contraindications: restlessness or agitation, hypertension, cardiovascular disease
5. Precautions: advanced age or debilitation
6. Drug interactions
   a) Tricyclic antidepressants: arrhythmias, tachycardia, hypertension
   b) Beta-blockers: hypertension, bradycardia, heart block
   c) Other CNS stimulants: increased cardiovascular effects, nervousness, insomnia, convulsions
   d) Digitalis glycosides: cardiac dysrhythmias
   e) MAO inhibitors: cardiac dysrhythmias, severe hypertension
   f) Thyroid hormones: enhancement of both agents' effects

C. Other central nervous system stimulants
1. Examples: doxapram (Dopram), methylphenidate (Ritalin)
2. Use/mechanism of action: treat respiratory depression due to drug overdose, disease, or anesthesia (doxapram); treat attention deficit disorder and narcolepsy by increasing excitatory CNS neurotransmitter activity, blocking inhibitory impulses or otherwise altering neurotransmitter availability and neuronal response
3. Adverse effects
   a) Doxapram: difficult urination, headache, diarrhea, dizziness, hiccups, cough, confusion, hypertension, dysrhythmias, dyspnea, convulsions, spasticity
   b) Methylphenidate, pemoline: anorexia, nervousness, insomnia, hypertension, tachycardia
4. Contraindications
   a) Doxapram: epilepsy, seizures, agitation, head injury, cerebral vascular accidents; newborn status
   b) Methylphenidate: glaucoma, agitation, depression, fatigue
5. Precautions
   a) Doxapram: hypertension
   b) Methylphenidate: epilepsy, hypertension, pregnancy, lactation
6. Drug interactions
   a) Doxapram: enhanced hypertensive effects with MAO inhibitors
   b) Methylphenidate
      (1) Other CNS stimulants: additive effects
      (2) MAO inhibitors: hypertensive crisis

D. Methylxanthines
1. Examples: caffeine, theophylline, theobromine
2. Use/mechanism of action: treat drowsiness; treat migraine (when used as adjunct to analgesics to relieve pain) by increasing excitatory CNS neurotransmitter activity, blocking inhibitory impulses or otherwise altering neurotransmitter availability and neuronal response
3. Adverse effects: nervousness, GI irritation
4. Contraindications: peptic ulcers, known hypersensitivity
5. Precautions: pregnancy, cardiac dysrhythmias
6. Drug interactions
   a) Other CNS stimulants: increased stimulant effects at very high doses
   b) MAO inhibitors: increased hypertensive effects

E. Nursing diagnoses
1. Sensory alterations (visual) related to blurred vision caused by amphetamine
2. Altered nutrition, less than body requirements, related to anorexia caused by CNS stimulant
3. Altered comfort related to dry mouth caused by CNS stimulant
4. Altered thought patterns related to agitation and irritability caused by CNS stimulant

F. Nursing implementation factors
1. Administration procedures
   a) Refrain from administering anorexiants to client who has been taking MAO inhibitors until a 2-week washout period has elapsed.
   b) Administer CNS stimulants in the morning to avoid insomnia.
   c) Avoid withdrawal symptoms by tapering amphetamine doses, not stopping them abruptly.
   d) Adjust doxapram infusion rate according to pulse, blood pressure, and deep tendon reflexes; monitor throughout infusion.
2. Daily monitoring and measurements
   a) Check blood and urine glucose levels in a diabetic client receiving anorexiant therapy.
   b) Monitor pulse and blood pressure of clients taking amphetamines.
   c) Measure arterial blood gases before administering doxapram and throughout infusion.
3. Points for client teaching
   a) Warn clients taking anorexiants that their coordination and alertness may be impaired.
   b) Suggest that clients taking anorexiants or amphetamines reduce dry mouth with ice chips or sugarless gum and candy.

     c) Caution clients that most CNS stimulants have a narrow therapeutic range and are generally for short-term use only.

     d) Warn clients of the risk of dependence and tell them not to change their dosage.

G. Nursing evaluations
1. Client maintains normal body weight and appetite.
2. Client's visual acuity remains normal.
3. Client relieves dry mouth with sugarless candy and gum.
4. Client maintains normal mental functioning and mood.

XI. Skeletal muscle relaxants

A. Examples: carisoprodol (Soma); chlorphenesin (Maolate); chlorzoxazone (Paraflex); cyclobenzaprine (Flexeril); metaxalone (Skelaxin); methocarbamol (Robaxin); orphenadrine (Norflex, Norgesic); dantrolene (Dantrium); diazepam (Valium); baclofen (Lioresal)

B. Use/mechanism of action: treat acute musculoskeletal pain and muscle spasticity associated with multiple sclerosis, cerebral palsy, cerebrovascular accidents, and spinal cord injury by causing CNS depression, acting directly on muscle to inhibit calcium ion release, acting on spinal cord, or enhancing inhibitory action of GABA (gamma-aminobutyric acid)

C. Adverse effects: drowsiness, dizziness, GI distress, ataxia, hypotension, blurred vision, bradycardia, urine retention, physical and psychologic dependence (with prolonged use), muscle weakness, depressed liver function, headache, confusion, nausea, fatigue, vertigo, hypotonia, muscle weakness, hallucinations, euphoria, depression, anxiety

D. Contraindications: pregnancy, lactation, hepatic disease

E. Precautions: hepatic, renal, cardiac, pulmonary impairment, brain disorders

F. Drug interactions
1. Alcohol, narcotics, barbiturates, anticonvulsants, tricyclic antidepressants, antianxiolytics: increased CNS effects, motor skill impairment, and respiratory depression caused by skeletal muscle relaxants
2. Cyclobenzaprine and MAO inhibitors: hyperpyrexia, excitation, seizures
3. Cyclobenzaprine and orphenadrine: increased adverse effects of cholinergic blockers

G. Nursing diagnoses
1. Pain related to adverse CNS effects
2. Impaired adjustment related to physical and psychologic dependence
3. Potential for injury related to CNS effects
4. Impaired physical mobility related to flaccid paralysis
5. Sensory-perceptual alteration related to adverse CNS effects

H. Nursing implementation factors
   1. Administration procedures
      a) Reduce baclofen dosage gradually, since abrupt withdrawal is associated with confusion, hallucinations, nightmares, paranoia, and rebound spasticity.
      b) Observe client who has received parenteral diazepam closely and ensure that he/she stays in bed for 3 hours.
   2. Daily monitoring and measurements
      a) All skeletal muscle relaxants
         (1) Monitor neuromuscular status.
         (2) Check bowel and bladder function.
         (3) Measure liver and kidney function.
      b) Baclofen: Monitor blood glucose levels in clients with diabetes.
   3. Points for client teaching
      a) Caution client receiving skeletal muscle relaxants that mental alertness may be impaired.
      b) Advise client receiving baclofen that maximum benefit may not be attained for 1–2 months.
      c) Warn female client of childbearing age that diazepam crosses the placental barrier and is associated with cleft lip.

I. Nursing evaluations
   1. Client reports increase in comfort and ability to perform activities of daily living.
   2. Client maintains normal mental functioning and mood.

1. To promote excretion of inhalation anesthetics after surgery, the nurse should:
   a. Administer a laxative.
   b. Force fluids.
   c. Encourage deep breathing.
   d. Suction respiratory secretions frequently.

2. Mrs. Delano still has not voided 6 hours after abdominal surgery, during which she received both inhalation and injected anesthetics. She denies any urge to urinate. Which action should the nurse take first?
   a. Assist Mrs. Delano to the bedside commode and provide privacy.
   b. Palpate Mrs. Delano's abdomen for suprapubic distention.
   c. Consult the physician for an order to catheterize Mrs. Delano.
   d. Increase the flow rate of Mrs. Delano's IV for 30 minutes.

3. Mrs. Chen has an order for meperidine (Demerol) 75 mg IV every 4 hours PRN for incisional pain. Four hours postoperatively she requests pain medication. Which of the following assessment findings should alert the nurse to consult the physician before administering the meperidine?
   a. Respiratory rate 9/minute
   b. Pulse 60 beats/minute
   c. Urine output 100 ml in the past 4 hours
   d. Bowel sounds hypoactive

4. Mr. Murphy, an 85-year-old with diabetes and hypertension, has developed osteoarthritis in both hips. Ibuprofen (Motrin) 200 mg QID is prescribed to control his arthritic pain. Which daily assessment will be most important for Mr. Murphy?
   a. Monitoring respiratory rate
   b. Testing for hearing loss
   c. Observing skin color
   d. Palpating for pedal edema

5. The client given a prescription for pilocarpine to treat glaucoma should be warned of potential problems with:
   a. Reading.
   b. Driving at night.
   c. Nasal congestion.
   d. Nosebleeds.

6. An appropriate nursing diagnosis for a client receiving dicyclomine (Bentyl) to treat irritable bowel syndrome would be:
   a. High risk for hyperthermia related to decreased perspiration.
   b. Diarrhea related to increased intestinal motility.
   c. Urge incontinence related to increased bladder muscle tone.
   d. Ineffective airway clearance related to increased respiratory secretions.

7. Oral albuterol (Proventil) 2 mg TID is prescribed for Mr. Rivoli to prevent bronchospasms due to asthma. Which advice regarding the scheduling of medication doses should the nurse give him?
   a. Take Proventil at least 1 hour after a meal.
   b. Take Proventil 2 hours after a meal.
   c. Take Proventil with a meal or snack.
   d. Do not take Proventil within 2 hours of bedtime.

8. Angela D'Amico is taking ergotamine tartrate (Ergomar) to control migraine headaches. She tells the nurse that her fingers feel "like they're asleep." The nurse should:
   a. Assess for factors that interfere with drug absorption.
   b. Consult the physician for an increase in drug dosage.
   c. Suggest warm hand soaks to control this side effect.
   d. Withhold the drug and report this symptom to the physician.

9. Mr. Smith is receiving atenolol (Tenormin) to manage his high blood pressure. Before his 10:00 A.M. dose, his apical rate is 54. The nurse should:

   a. Administer the ordered dose.
   b. Administer half of the ordered dose.
   c. Discontinue the drug.
   d. Notify the physician of the pulse before giving the dose.

10. Eight-year-old Ricky Graham is being treated for attention deficit disorder with methylphenidate (Ritalin). He needs to be monitored for:

    a. Weight gain.
    b. Growth retardation.
    c. Swallowing problems.
    d. Habituation to the drug.

11. The client for whom phenytoin (Dilantin) is prescribed to control seizures should be taught to:

    a. Brush the teeth 3–4 times daily.
    b. Avoid milk and dairy products.
    c. Massage the scalp gently at least once a day.
    d. Consume at least 3000 ml/day of fluid.

12. Benztropine mesylate (Cogentin) is often prescribed to prevent or control extrapyramidal side effects of other drugs. To evaluate the effectiveness of this therapy, the nurse should assess for:

    a. Irregular cardiac rhythms.
    b. Sleep disturbances.
    c. Abnormal movements.
    d. Confusion or disorientation.

ANSWERS

1. **Correct answer is c.** Inhalation anesthetics are excreted by the lungs in exhaled air. Deep-breathing speeds excretion by increasing exhaled air volume.

   a. Laxatives would speed excretion of drugs via the intestinal tract. This is not the route of excretion for inhaled anesthetics.

   b. Forcing fluids would promote renal excretion. Inhaled anesthetics are not excreted by this route.

   d. The lungs are the route of excretion for anesthetics, but they are excreted in the exhaled gases, not secretions.

2. **Correct answer is b.** Urine retention is a common side effect of anesthetics, but failure to void in the early postoperative period can also be caused by decreased production of urine, due to fluid shifts and anesthesia effects. To determine whether urine retention is the problem, the nurse should palpate for a full bladder.

   a. If a full bladder is first identified, assisting client to the bedside commode might be the second action. Mrs. Delano should not be left alone in a sitting position, since syncope can occur after anesthesia.

   c. Requesting an order for catheterization is premature. Assessment should come first. Efforts to stimulate voiding, such as assuming a sitting position, listening to the sound of running water, or placing the hand in warm water, may be effective and prevent the need for more invasive procedures.

   d. Increasing the IV rate would require a physician's order. If the problem is urine retention, increasing urine formation will further distend the bladder.

3. **Correct answer is a.** Respiratory depression is a common side effect with short-term use of narcotics, especially during the period of recovery from anesthesia. If the respiratory rate is less than 10/minute, the physician should be consulted about whether the ordered dose should be reduced or withheld. Administering the narcotic could further depress respirations or cause respiratory arrest.

   b. A pulse rate of 60 beats/minute is within normal limits.

   c. Urine output is often low postoperatively due to fluid shifts during surgery. Since pain will interfere with voiding and add to surgical stress, analgesics would not normally be withheld.

d. Anesthesia and surgery often depress intestinal function, so hypoactive bowel sounds would not be an abnormal finding. The narcotic would not be withheld for this reason.

4. **Correct answer is d.** Nonsteroidal anti-inflammatory drugs (NSAIDs) such as ibuprofen may cause sodium and fluid retention, especially in clients with high blood pressure or congestive heart failure, who are predisposed to the problem. Pedal edema is a sign of fluid retention.

    a. Respiratory depression is a problem with narcotics, not with NSAIDs.
    b. The ears may be affected by NSAID toxicity, although this is more common with aspirin. This toxicity produces tinnitus, not hearing loss.
    c. Observing skin color would be appropriate with prolonged or frequent use of acetaminophen (Tylenol), which can damage the liver. Jaundice would appear as a sign of hepatotoxicity. This is not a common problem with NSAIDs, although cyanosis may appear as a late sign of respiratory depression (see answer a).

5. **Correct answer is b.** Pilocarpine produces pupil constriction and impairs accommodation for distant vision. The pupils may not dilate sufficiently to make use of the dim light available at night, making driving difficult.

    a. Since the pupils are constricted with this drug, near vision, including the ability to read, is not impaired. Any blurring that occurs affects distant vision, which requires pupil dilation.
    c and d. If precautions are not taken to prevent drops from draining through the nasolacrimal duct onto nasal mucous membranes, the drug may be absorbed into systemic circulation and systemic side effects may occur. Nasal congestion and bleeding are not anticipated side effects of cholinergic drugs.

6. **Correct answer is a.** Anticholinergics decrease perspiration, resulting in decreased ability to lose heat. The risk of heat illness, such as heat exhaustion or heatstroke, is increased.

    b. Anticholinergics decrease intestinal motility and reduce colon spasms. Constipation is the most likely gastrointestinal side effect.
    c. Urinary retention is the common side effect with anticholinergic drugs. Urgency or urge incontinence may occur with cholinergics.
    d. Anticholinergics decrease respiratory secretions.

7. **Correct answer is c.** Adrenergic drugs often cause nausea and even vomiting. To prevent GI upset, these medications should be taken with food unless ordered otherwise.

    a and b. Taking albuterol 1 or 2 hours after a meal ensures that the medication is taken on an empty stomach, increasing the risk of nausea and vomiting.
    d. Although not taking albuterol within 2 hours of bedtime would decrease the chance of sleep disturbance, it would not provide for symptom control during sleep. Since clients with respiratory problems often experience symptoms at night, a bedtime dose may be important.

8. **Correct answer is d.** This is an early sign of ergotism, which reflects toxicity of ergot-derivative drugs. The drug should be withheld until the client can be evaluated by a physician.

    a. Ergotism results from drug levels that are too high. Impaired absorption would lower drug levels.
    b. Since finger numbness is a symptom of drug toxicity, a dosage increase would be inappropriate.
    c. Warm soaks might be prescribed to improve circulation to her hands, but since this is a sign of toxicity, answer d is more appropriate.

9. Correct answer is d. Bradycardia is a possibly serious side effect of beta-adrenergic blocking drugs. The physician may reduce the dose to avoid worsening the bradycardia.

a. Administering the usual dosage may worsen the bradycardia, reducing tissue perfusion below adequate levels.

b. Altering drug dosage is not a nursing measure. A physician's order would be required.

c. Abruptly discontinuing a beta-adrenergic blocker can lead to rebound hypertension, myocardial infarction, or arrhythmia. Discontinuing the drug without consulting the physician would be inappropriate.

10. Correct answer is b. Growth retardation is a common effect of methylphenidate. Records of height and weight should be kept. Drug holidays help reduce this effect.

a. Weight loss is usually due to the appetite suppressant effects of psychomotor stimulants.

c. Psychomotor stimulants are not known to cause problems with swallowing.

d. Habituation to psychomotor stimulants does not occur in children being treated for attention deficit disorder, although it would be a concern in adults who are being treated for other problems.

11. Correct answer is a. Frequent oral hygiene delays development of gingival hyperplasia.

b. Since phenytoin antagonizes vitamin D and decreases intestinal absorption of calcium, increased intake of milk would be desirable.

c. Massaging the scalp is often suggested to reduce hair loss. Since hirsutism (excessive hair growth) is a side effect of phenytoin, it would be irrelevant.

d. Forcing fluids would be indicated to prevent dehydration or decrease the risk of renal toxicity. These are not anticipated effects of phenytoin.

12. Correct answer is c. The extrapyramidal system controls muscle movement. Antipsychotic drugs often cause Parkinson's syndrome or abnormal muscle movements. Antiparkinson drugs, such as benztropine, are given to prevent these effects.

a and d. The extrapyramidal system is not related to irregular cardiac rhythms, confusion, or disorientation. Because antiparkinson drugs can cause these problems, they would not be useful in treating them.

b. Sleep disturbances are not related to the extrapyramidal system. Antiparkinson drugs have no beneficial effect on sleep disorders.

4

Drugs Affecting Mental Functioning

NURSING HIGHLIGHTS

1. The goal in caring for psychiatric clients is to obtain therapeutic results on as low a maintenance dose as possible. The nurse can help by being a careful observer of changes in client's behavior and affect.
2. Because psychotropic medications are often administered long-term, it is vital to assess the client often and carefully for adverse effects.
3. The nurse should be sensitive to small changes in mouth, tongue, and facial movements that might be the first signs of tardive dyskinesia caused by neuroleptic therapy.
4. A drug holiday is not a holiday for the nurse! Adverse effects such as tardive dyskinesia may first appear during these drug-free periods.

GLOSSARY

affective disorder—a mood disturbance, including depression, anxiety, mania, and elation

anxiolytic—a drug that alleviates anxiety, such as a sedative or tranquilizer

barbiturate—a salt or derivative of barbituric acid used for its sedative and hypnotic effects

chorea—recurring jerky, rapid, involuntary movements

extrapyramidal symptoms—movement disorders, including akathisia, akinesia, dystonia, and parkinsonian movements, that are caused by centrally acting antidopaminergic drugs

hypnotic—a sleep-inducing agent

Tourette's syndrome—a neurologic disorder that often presents in childhood as blinking and facial grimaces and may later include barking, grunting, movement disorders, and shouting

ENHANCED OUTLINE

See text pages
_____

I. Sedative, hypnotic, and anxiolytic agents

A. Benzodiazepines
   1. Examples: flurazepam (Dalmane), lorazepam (Ativan), quazepam (Doral), temazepam (Restoril), triazolam (Halcion), alprazolam (Xanax), diazepam (Valium)
   2. Use/mechanism of action: sedate or calm client or induce sleep as a treatment for insomnia by increasing effect of inhibitory neurotransmitter GABA (gamma-aminobutyric acid)
   3. Adverse effects: daytime sedation, hangover effect, dose-related dizziness; occasional fatigue, dry mouth, muscle weakness, nausea, respiratory depression; physical and psychologic dependence with prolonged high-dose use
   4. Contraindications: impaired consciousness, respiratory depression, pregnancy, glaucoma
   5. Precautions: depression, renal or hepatic impairment, chronic pulmonary insufficiency, lactation
   6. Drug interactions
      a) Central nervous system (CNS) depressants: enhanced sedative and CNS depressant effects
      b) Cimetidine with flurazepam, quazepam, or triazolam: inhibition of metabolism, with increased sedation and CNS depression
      c) Oral contraceptives and flurazepam: increased sedation
      d) Oral contraceptives and lorazepam or temazepam: decreased sedation

B. Barbiturates
   1. Examples: amobarbital (Amytal); aprobarbital (Alurate); butabarbital (Butisol, Buticaps); mephobarbital (Mebaral); pentobarbital (Nembutal); phenobarbital (Luminal); secobarbital (Seconal)
   2. Use/mechanism of action: sedate or calm client or induce sleep as a treatment for insomnia or anxiety by acting as nonspecific CNS depressant
   3. Adverse effects: daytime sedation, hangover effect, dizziness, depression; impairment of judgment and motor skills during hangover; REM sleep rebound after discontinuation; tolerance, psychologic and physical dependence with prolonged use
   4. Contraindications: impaired consciousness, respiratory depression, porphyria, pregnancy, nephritis, renal disease, prodromal signs of hepatic coma
   5. Precautions: lactation, depression, hepatic damage, history of drug abuse
   6. Drug interactions
      a) Hydantoins, valproic acid, and chloramphenicol: inhibition of phenobarbital metabolism, increasing risk of toxicity
      b) Beta-blockers: stimulation of beta-blocker metabolism, decreasing effectiveness
      c) Chloramphenicol, corticosteroids, doxycycline, oral anticoagulants, oral contraceptives, quinidine, tricyclic antidepressants, metronidazole, digitoxin, theophylline, cyclosporine: reduced effectiveness because of induction of metabolism by barbiturates

C. Miscellaneous agents
   1. Examples: chloral hydrate (Noctec), ethchlorvynol (Placidyl), glutethimide (Doriden), methyprylon (Noludar), paraldehyde (Paral), buspirone (BuSpar)
   2. Use/mechanism of action: sedate or calm client or induce sleep as a treatment for insomnia or anxiety by exercising CNS depressant effects similar to those of barbiturates
   3. Adverse effects: gastrointestinal (GI) irritation, limited hangover effect; respiratory depression, respiratory failure at high doses; tolerance, psychologic and physical dependence with prolonged use
   4. Contraindications: impaired consciousness, respiratory depression, renal dysfunction, gastroenteritis, ulcers, porphyria
   5. Precautions: lactation, depression, hepatic damage, history of drug abuse
   6. Drug interactions
      a) Other CNS depressants: increased CNS depression
      b) Chloral hydrate and oral anticoagulants: increased bleeding
      c) Paraldehyde and disulfiram: increased CNS depression; disulfiram toxicity, including respiratory depression, cardiac arrhythmias, seizures, and unconsciousness
      d) Oral anticoagulants and glutethimide or ethchlorvynol: increased risk of blood clots

D. Nursing diagnoses
1. Altered role performance related to dependence on sedative, hypnotic, or anxiolytic agent
2. Impaired gas exchange related to respiratory depression
3. Potential for injury related to impaired judgment and motor skills
4. Sleep pattern disturbance related to rebound insomnia
5. Ineffective coping related to impaired judgment
6. Impaired home maintenance management related to dependence on sedative, hypnotic, or anxiolytic agent

E. Nursing implementation factors
1. Administration procedures
   a) Keep epinephrine and corticosteroids at hand in case of hypersensitivity reactions.
   b) Watch client take medication to deter drug hoarding.
   c) Fit drug administration or monitoring into client's daily routine rather than waking him/her.
   d) Rotate ampule rather than shaking it when preparing to administer amobarbital; mix with sterile water only.
   e) Refrain from using a cloudy solution of phenobarbital, secobarbital, or pentobarbital; do not mix other drugs in same syringe.
   f) Avoid using intramuscular (IM) route for barbiturates; select a large muscle mass if IM administration is necessary.
   g) Give chloral hydrate orally with food to reduce GI irritation.
2. Daily monitoring and measurements
   a) Monitor and document mental status.
   b) Monitor vital signs, paying special attention to signs of respiratory depression.
   c) Make respiratory assessment before and after drug administration.
   d) Measure fluid intake and output.
3. Points for client teaching
   a) Advise client with insomnia to try other measures before taking prescribed hypnotic (e.g., warm shower or bath, glass of warm milk, elimination of daytime naps, relaxation techniques).
   b) Warn client and family to beware of dizziness and falls; client should not drive or use machinery until drug's effects on balance and alertness have been established.
   c) Warn client not to discontinue medication abruptly without consulting physician.
   d) Tell client not to give drug to friends or family members.
   e) Warn client not to drink alcohol during CNS depressant therapy because of danger of fatal respiratory depression.

F. Nursing evaluations
   1. Client shows no signs of dependence.
   2. Client maintains normal respiratory rate and pattern.
   3. Client avoids drug hangover.
   4. Client discontinues drug slowly, avoiding rebound effect.

II. Antidepressant and mood disorder drugs

See text pages
_____

A. Tricyclic antidepressants
   1. Examples: amitriptyline (Elavil); desipramine (Norpramin); imipramine (Tofranil); nortriptyline (Aventyl, Pamelor); protriptyline (Vivactil)
   2. Use/mechanism of action: treat affective disorders, including depression and bipolar disorder (manic-depressive illness), probably by increasing receptor sensitivity to serotonin and/or norepinephrine
   3. Adverse effects: anticholinergic effects (dry mouth, blurred vision, urine retention, constipation), orthostatic hypotension, hypertension, tachycardia, anxiety, ataxia, sedation, confusion, insomnia, headache, dizziness, extrapyramidal symptoms, anorexia, increased appetite, weight gain, abdominal cramps, photosensitivity, agranulocytosis, prostatic hypertrophy; seizures (rare)
   4. Contraindications: urine retention, glaucoma
   5. Precautions: pregnancy, lactation, suicidal tendencies, cardiovascular disease, liver impairment
   6. Drug interactions
      a) Amphetamines, sympathomimetics: increased catecholamine release, hypertension
      b) Barbiturates: decreased serum antidepressant levels
      c) MAO (monoamine oxidase) inhibitors: hyperpyrexia, excitation, seizures
      d) Anticholinergics: increased anticholinergic effects
      e) Clonidine, guanethidine: reduced antihypertensive effect
      f) Cimetidine: impaired liver metabolism of antidepressants, causing possible toxicity

B. MAO (monoamine oxidase) inhibitors
   1. Examples: isocarboxazid (Marplan), phenelzine (Nardil), tranylcypromine (Parnate)
   2. Use/mechanism of action: treat affective disorders, including depression and bipolar disorder, by inhibiting MAO, the enzyme that metabolizes the neurotransmitters norepinephrine and serotonin, thus increasing their availability
   3. Adverse effects: restlessness, drowsiness, dizziness, headache, nausea, dry mouth, blurred vision, orthostatic hypotension; hypertensive crisis (rare)
   4. Contraindications: cardiovascular disease, pheochromocytoma, known hypersensitivity
   5. Precautions: diabetes, epilepsy, pregnancy, lactation

6. Drug interactions
    a) Amphetamines, sympathomimetics, nonamphetamine antianorexia agents: increased catecholamine release, hypertension
    b) Tricyclic antidepressants, fluoxetine, cyclobenzaprine: hyperpyrexia, excitation, seizures
    c) Doxapram: hypertension, arrhythmias; potentiation of doxapram's adverse effects
    d) Levodopa: hypertension
    e) Hypoglycemic agents: hypoglycemia
    f) Meperidine: excitation, hypotension or hypertension, hyperpyrexia, coma
    g) Tyramine-rich foods, including aged cheese, sour cream, yogurt, beer, wine, chocolate, licorice, soy sauce, and yeast: hypertensive crisis

C. Second-generation antidepressants
    1. Examples: fluoxetine (Prozac), trazodone (Desyrel)
    2. Use/mechanism of action: treat affective disorders, including depression and bipolar disorder, by inhibiting reuptake of serotonin
    3. Adverse effects: headache, nervousness, anxiety, insomnia, nausea, anorexia, sedation, dizziness
    4. Contraindications: acute recovery period after myocardial infarction
    5. Precautions: cardiac disease, pregnancy, lactation
    6. Drug interactions
        a) Fluoxetine and diazepam: increased half-life of diazepam
        b) Fluoxetine and MAO inhibitors: seizures
        c) Trazodone and phenytoin: increased phenytoin levels
        d) Trazodone: additive effects with CNS depressants and antihypertensives

D. Lithium
    1. Example: lithium
    2. Use/mechanism of action: treat affective disorders, including depression and bipolar disorder, probably by normalizing catecholamine receptor activity by increasing norepinephrine and serotonin uptake
    3. Adverse effects: nausea, vomiting, tremor, polydipsia, polyuria
    4. Contraindications: epilepsy, renal disease, cardiovascular disease, severe dehydration, sodium depletion, pregnancy, lactation
    5. Precautions: thyroid disease
    6. Drug interactions
        a) Diuretics, low-salt diets: increased lithium levels
        b) Nonsteroidal anti-inflammatory drugs (NSAIDs): inhibition of lithium excretion
        c) Potassium iodide: hypothyroidism

         d) High salt intake, sodium bicarbonate, theophylline: decreased lithium levels

         e) Phenothiazines, carbamazepine: neurotoxicity

E. Nursing diagnoses
1. Potential for injury related to hypertensive crisis (MAO inhibitor)
2. Sensory-perceptual alteration related to blurred vision or photosensitivity (tricyclic antidepressant or MAO inhibitor)
3. Urinary retention related to receptor modification (tricyclic antidepressant)
4. Potential for injury related to seizures
5. Constipation related to anticholinergic effect
6. Potential for injury related to tremor (lithium)
7. Altered role performance related to benzodiazepine or barbiturate dependence
8. Pain related to headache
9. Ineffective individual coping related to benzodiazepine or barbiturate dependence

F. Nursing implementation factors
1. Administration procedures
    a) Change antidepressant administration time to early evening or morning, respectively, if drowsiness or insomnia occurs as a side effect.
    b) Do not stop tranylcypromine abruptly, but taper off dosage over a 2-week period to prevent withdrawal reactions.
    c) Be prepared to prevent client from falling if orthostatic hypotension or dizziness occurs.
    d) Administer lithium with food to reduce GI effects.
2. Daily monitoring and measurements
    a) Monitor client receiving MAO inhibitor for signs of hypertensive crisis, including increased blood pressure, severe headache, neck stiffness, palpitations.
    b) Monitor client for suicidal tendencies.
    c) Assess client for constipation resulting from tricyclic antidepressant use.
    d) Record fluid intake and output.
    e) Inform physician and withhold fluoxetine if client develops rash.
    f) Monitor client who is taking lithium and who has polyuria or diabetes insipidus for signs of dehydration.
    g) Monitor client's lithium level, being aware that a concentration over 1.5 mEq/L may cause toxicity.
    h) Monitor white blood cell count (WBC) of client taking lithium.
3. Points for client teaching
    a) Ensure that a client receiving an MAO inhibitor knows the foods that interact dangerously with the drug, including aged cheese, sour cream, yogurt, beer, wine, chocolate, licorice, soy sauce, and yeast; frequently review this material.
    b) Teach client and family to recognize the signs of hypertensive crisis.

c) Instruct client to recognize and report urine retention.
d) Tell male clients that drug-induced impotence may occur with an MAO inhibitor and some tricyclic antidepressants but that condition will resolve when drug is discontinued.
e) Caution client receiving an antidepressant to rise slowly to reduce the effects of orthostatic hypotension.
f) Warn client not to drive or operate dangerous machinery until response is established.
g) Explain to client that full response may take several weeks.
h) Instruct clients to take their antidepressants with food to enhance absorption and reduce dizziness.
i) Teach client and family to recognize signs of lithium toxicity, including confusion, lethargy, hyperreflexia, and seizures.
j) Advise client that tremor may occur with lithium therapy but that it will stop when therapy is discontinued.

G. Nursing evaluations
1. Client reports improved sense of well-being, improved coping, sleeping, appetite, and energy level.
2. Client's blood pressure remains normal.
3. Client has no adverse reactions to drug.
4. Side effects diminish to tolerable levels and therapeutic effect is sustained when dosage is reduced.
5. Client maintains normal fluid balance.
6. Client shows no sign of benzodiazepine or barbiturate dependence.

III. Antipsychotic drugs (neuroleptics)

See text pages
_____

A. Phenothiazines
1. Examples: chlorpromazine (Thorazine), trifluoperazine (Stelazine), thioridazine (Mellaril)
2. Use/mechanism of action: control psychotic symptoms, treat Tourette's syndrome and Huntington's chorea by blocking dopamine receptors in the limbic system, hypothalamus, and/or other regions of the brain
3. Adverse effects (see Nurse Alert, "Serious Adverse Effects of Neuroleptic Drugs")
   a) Extrapyramidal symptoms, including dystonia, akathisia, pseudoparkinsonism, tardive dyskinesia (see Nurse Alert, "Tardive Dyskinesia")
   b) Hypotension, sedation, seizures
   c) Neuroleptic malignant syndrome (fever, tachycardia, tachypnea, diaphoresis)
4. Contraindications: coma, pregnancy, lactation, blood dyscrasia, liver damage, known hypersensitivity, CNS depression, Parkinson's disease, prostate hypertrophy, urinary obstruction

5. Precautions: cardiovascular, hepatic, or chronic respiratory disease, suicidal tendencies
6. Drug interactions
   a) Guanethidine: inhibition of guanethidine uptake, reducing effectiveness
   b) CNS depressants: increased CNS depression; decreased phenothiazine effectiveness
   c) Anticholinergics: increased anticholinergic effects; decreased phenothiazine effectiveness
   d) Amphetamines and nonamphetamine antianorexia agents: mutual inhibition
   e) Levodopa: reduced antiparkinsonian effects of levodopa
   f) Droperidol: increased risk of extrapyramidal effects
   g) Anticonvulsants: lowered seizure threshold
   h) Tricyclic depressants, beta-blockers: increased serum levels for both classes of drugs
   i) Lithium: increased risk of lithium toxicity

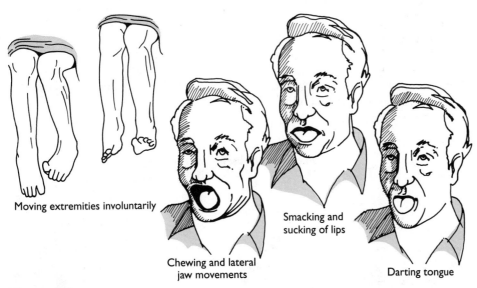

Moving extremities involuntarily

Chewing and lateral jaw movements

Smacking and sucking of lips

Darting tongue

Figure 4–1
Signs of Tardive Dyskinesia

B. Other agents
   1. Examples: clozapine (Clozaril), haloperidol (Haldol)
   2. Use/mechanism of action: control psychotic symptoms, treat Tourette's syndrome and Huntington's chorea by blocking dopamine receptors in the limbic system, hypothalamus, and/or other regions of the brain
   3. Adverse effects
      a) Extrapyramidal symptoms, including dystonia, akathisia, pseudo-parkinsonism, tardive dyskinesia (see Nurse Alert, "Tardive Dyskinesia")
      b) Hypotension, sedation, seizures
      c) Neutropenia or agranulocytosis with clozapine
   4. Contraindications: coma, pregnancy, lactation, blood dyscrasia, liver damage, known hypersensitivity, CNS depression, Parkinson's disease, prostate hypertrophy, urinary obstruction
   5. Precautions: cardiovascular, hepatic, or chronic respiratory disease, suicidal tendencies
   6. Drug interactions
      a) Haloperidol and lithium: increased risk of lithium toxicity
      b) Clozapine
         (1) Anticholinergics: increased anticholinergic effects
         (2) Antihypertensives: increased hypotensive effects
         (3) Other CNS drugs: additive CNS effects
         (4) Bone marrow suppressants: increased risk of agranulocytosis

C. Nursing diagnoses
   1. Potential for injury related to extrapyramidal effects
   2. Potential for urinary retention related to extrapyramidal effects
   3. Potential for constipation related to extrapyramidal effects
   4. Potential for altered thought processes related to extrapyramidal effects
   5. Impaired physical mobility related to extrapyramidal effects of antipsychotic agent

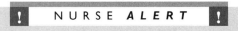

! NURSE *ALERT* !

Tardive Dyskinesia

Tardive dyskinesia is an irreversible adverse effect of neuroleptic drugs. Everyone caring for a client on neuroleptic medication must be alert for subtle early signs of this condition, such as lip smacking, fine wormlike tongue movements, and involuntary movements in the arms and legs.

6. Hyperthermia related to neuroleptic malignant syndrome caused by antipsychotic agent

D. Nursing implementation factors
   1. Administration procedures
      a) Refrain from discontinuing drug abruptly when a drug holiday is prescribed.
      b) Avoid administering haloperidol intravenously (IV).
      c) Be sure oral (PO) doses are swallowed, not hoarded.
   2. Daily monitoring and measurements
      a) Observe and report client behavior carefully.
      b) Watch client for extrapyramidal symptoms, such as slow involuntary movements of arms and legs and abnormal mouth movements.
      c) Monitor client receiving phenothiazines and CNS depressants for signs of respiratory depression.
      d) Monitor blood pressure; review lab tests for signs of hematologic or hepatic abnormalities and intake and output.
   3. Points for client teaching
      a) Teach client to reduce dry mouth impact of anticholinergic effects by chewing sugarless gum and increasing fluid intake.
      b) Inform family that normalization of symptoms may not occur for several weeks after beginning antipsychotic therapy.
      c) Stress importance of taking drug exactly as prescribed and not reducing dosage without consulting physician.
      d) Teach family members the signs of tardive dyskinesia and other extrapyramidal effects; have them report symptoms to physician immediately.

E. Nursing evaluations
   1. Client demonstrates better reality orientation and social interaction and decreased agitation.
   2. Client has no extrapyramidal symptoms.
   3. Client has no symptoms of neuroleptic malignant syndrome.

1. Seventy-year-old Mrs. Quigley received temazepam (Restoril) 15 mg at 10:00 P.M. When she awakens at 5:00 A.M., she is confused and agitated. The nurse should:

   a. Apply a soft waist restraint to prevent injury.
   b. Administer a second dose of temazepam (according to PRN order).
   c. Hold Mrs. Quigley's hand and talk quietly to her.
   d. Consult the physician about ordering a different sedative medication.

2. Lorazepam (Ativan) 2 mg is prescribed for 24-year-old Tasha Long to manage anxiety. Tasha has been taking oral contraceptives for 2 years. The nurse should anticipate which of the following as a result of the interaction between these 2 drugs?

   a. Breakthrough bleeding
   b. Excessive sedation
   c. Decreased sedation
   d. Increased risk of hepatotoxicity

3. Mrs. Fisher has received pentobarbital (Nembutal) to help her sleep at night during her first 3 postoperative days in the hospital. She will not be taking it after discharge. Which information about barbiturate effects should the nurse include in Mrs. Fisher's discharge teaching?

   a. She may have unusually vivid dreams for 2–3 nights.
   b. She may experience some anxiety due to withdrawal of the drug.
   c. She may feel fatigued or drowsy for 48 hours, until the drug is completely eliminated.
   d. She should report any breathing difficulties to her physician.

4. Nancy Elliott is about to begin taking phenobarbital (Luminal) to treat a seizure disorder. Instructions provided to her about this therapy should include which of the following?

   a. See your dentist every 6 months to monitor for gingival hyperplasia.
   b. Avoid alcohol while taking phenobarbital.
   c. Notify your physician of any unintended weight loss over 5 lb.
   d. Use an electric razor and a soft toothbrush.

5. An appropriate nursing diagnosis for a client receiving tricyclic antidepressants (TCAs) would be:

   a. Potential for fluid volume deficit related to diuretic effects of medication.
   b. Constipation related to anticholinergic effects of medication.
   c. Urge incontinence related to cholinergic effects of medication.
   d. Ineffective breathing patterns related to CNS depressant effects of medication.

6. Marie Henley, who has been under treatment for depression, attempted suicide by taking her entire bottle of imipramine (Tofranil). While she is being treated for the overdose, it will be critical to monitor her for which toxic effect?

   a. Severe hypertension
   b. Respiratory arrest
   c. Acute renal failure
   d. Cardiac arrhythmias

7. Clients taking MAO (monoamine oxidase) inhibitors to relieve depression should be cautioned to avoid:

   a. Aged cheeses.
   b. Dark green leafy vegetables.
   c. Red meat.
   d. Dairy products.

8. Selena Jenkins, who is taking phenelzine (Nardil) to treat depression, drank several glasses of red wine with dinner. She has been admitted to the emergency room with a blood pressure of 214/112. The nurse should anticipate an order to administer:
   a. Phentolamine (Regitine).
   b. Neostigmine (Prostigmin).
   c. Acetylcysteine (Mucomyst).
   d. Atropine.

9. Mary, who is receiving trazodone (Desyrel) 50 mg TID for depression, complains of feeling dizzy after taking her medication. The nurse should first:
   a. Withhold the trazodone and notify the physician.
   b. Administer future doses with meals.
   c. Consult the physician for a dosage reduction.
   d. Increase Mary's fluid intake to 2000 ml/day.

10. Mark Avery, whose symptoms of bipolar disorder are controlled with lithium carbonate, needs a diagnostic x-ray for which the preparation is NPO overnight and enemas. Which nursing action is indicated?
    a. Tell Mark to increase his sodium intake the day before the test.
    b. Warn Mark that he should avoid hazardous activities during the preparation because he may experience muscle weakness.
    c. Inform the radiologist that Mark takes lithium before beginning the preparation.
    d. Monitor Mark for manic symptoms during the preparation.

11. An appropriate nursing diagnosis to address potential side effects of lithium therapy for the treatment of bipolar disorder would be:
    a. Constipation related to anticholinergic effects of the medication.
    b. Altered oral mucous membranes related to dry mouth.
    c. Sexual dysfunction related to decreased libido.
    d. Fluid volume deficit related to polyuria.

12. The client receiving phenothiazine antipsychotics should be taught to:
    a. Lie down for 1 hour after each dose to prevent hypotension.
    b. Take liquid medication through a straw to avoid discoloring the teeth.
    c. Avoid organ meats to prevent hypertensive crisis.
    d. Use strong sunblock and protective clothing when outdoors to prevent skin discoloration.

ANSWERS

1. **Correct answer is c.** A brief period of confusion and excitement upon awakening after use of a benzodiazepine hypnotic drug is not unusual, especially in the elderly. Touch, quiet speech, and reorientation to the environment should be adequate to manage it.

   a. Restraints are likely to increase Mrs. Quigley's anxiety and prolong her confused and agitated state.
   b. Temazepam is used only as a hypnotic. It would be inappropriate to administer it so close to the normal time of arising.
   d. Additional sedation is unnecessary and inappropriate at this time. If touching and talking quietly are ineffective, this might be an appropriate next step.

2. **Correct answer is c.** When oral contraceptives and lorazepam are given together, the sedative effect of lorazepam is reduced.

   a. Breakthrough bleeding would occur if the oral contraceptive's effects were decreased. Lorazepam does not decrease oral contraceptive effects.
   b. Increased sedation may occur if flurazepam (Dalmane) is given with oral contraceptives but does not occur with lorazepam.
   d. Hepatotoxicity is not a common problem with either drug and does not occur with the interaction.

3. Correct answer is a. REM rebound, which produces vivid and bizarre dreams, may occur even after a few days of barbiturate use.

b. Withdrawal symptoms would not appear until the client had been taking the drug long enough to produce physical dependence. Physical dependence develops after prolonged use.

c. Although there may be a hangover effect the morning after a dose is taken, these symptoms would not persist for 48 hours after the dose.

d. The instruction to report breathing problems would be given at the time the medication is administered. Respiratory depression would not occur this long after the drug was taken.

4. Correct answer is b. The combination of alcohol and a barbiturate can produce potentially fatal respiratory depression.

a. This precaution relates to phenytoin (Dilantin). Phenobarbital does not cause gingival hyperplasia.

c. This precaution applies to succinimide anticonvulsants. Weight loss is not a common side effect of phenobarbital.

d. Use of an electric razor and soft toothbrush applies to valproic acid. Inhibition of platelet aggregation is not a side effect of phenobarbital.

5. Correct answer is b. Tricyclic antidepressants (TCAs) have anticholinergic side effects, which include constipation.

a. TCAs have no diuretic effects.

c. TCAs have anticholinergic side effects. Urinary retention, not urge incontinence, would be expected.

d. TCAs do not have respiratory depressant effects.

6. Correct answer is d. At toxic levels, the tricyclic antidepressants (TCAs) commonly induce dangerous arrhythmias.

a. Orthostatic hypotension is a common side effect of TCAs. Hypertension would not be expected.

b. Respiratory depression is not a major effect of TCAs. Respiratory arrest is much more likely with CNS depressant drugs.

c. TCAs are not highly nephrotoxic. Although acute renal failure may occur with any overdose, it is not common with tricyclics.

7. Correct answer is a. High-tyramine foods, such as red wines, aged cheeses, smoked meats, and yeast extracts, can induce hypertensive crisis when they are taken with MAO inhibitors.

b, c, and **d.** Dark green leafy vegetables, red meat, and dairy products are not high in tyramine, so none would be expected to have a problematic interaction with MAO inhibitors.

8. Correct answer is a. The alpha-adrenergic blocker phentolamine is the treatment of choice for hypertensive crisis caused by interaction of MAO inhibitors with tyramine.

b. Neostigmine is the antagonist for neuromuscular blocking agents.

c. Acetylcysteine is the antagonist for acute acetaminophen overdose.

d. Atropine is the antagonist for anticholinesterase drugs. Given to someone taking MAO inhibitors, it could worsen the hypertensive response.

9. Correct answer is b. Administering trazodone with meals or at bedtime minimizes the dizziness and sedation that may occur as side effects.

a. Dizziness is a common side effect, not a sign of toxicity. There is no reason to withhold the drug when the symptom can probably be managed with appropriate interventions.

c. If the dizziness is too distressing for Mary and is not helped by giving trazodone with meals, dosage reduction would be appropriate. However, it is not the best initial choice.

d. Dizziness due to trazodone is related to CNS effects, not fluid imbalance. Forcing fluid is unlikely to relieve it.

10. **Correct answer is c.** Lithium has a narrow therapeutic range. Since adequate hydration is essential for lithium excretion, a dehydrating preparation puts Mark at risk for lithium toxicity. The radiologist may order an alteration in the preparation or initiate IV fluids to maintain Mark's usual sodium and fluid balance and prevent lithium toxicity during the preparation.

a. Increasing sodium intake can decrease serum lithium levels. The physician should be consulted before any alteration in sodium intake is made.
b. Muscle weakness would be a sign of lithium toxicity and should be reported to the physician. Simply avoiding hazardous activities would not be an adequate response.
d. The preparation is likely to increase serum lithium levels. Manic symptoms occur if serum lithium levels decrease, so this preparation is unlikely to cause them.

11. **Correct answer is d.** Polyuria often occurs in the first weeks of therapy and may result in fluid volume deficit if fluid intake is inadequate to replace lost fluid.

a. Constipation is a common side effect of tricyclic antidepressants (TCAs) but is unlikely with lithium. Diarrhea occurs with lithium toxicity.
b. Dry mouth is not a common side effect of lithium. It does occur with TCAs and antipsychotics.
c. Sexual dysfunction is not a common side effect of lithium. It is more likely to occur with TCAs or sedatives.

12. **Correct answer is d.** Photosensitivity is a common side effect. Exposure to sunlight can cause a purplish-brown skin discoloration.

a. Lying down after doses is indicated only with the first few doses, to prevent orthostatic hypotension. Thereafter, it is usually manageable by having the client change position slowly.
b. Liquid phenothiazines do not discolor teeth, although they may cause contact dermatitis if spilled on skin.
c. Clients on long-term phenothiazine therapy should actually increase intake of organ meats to provide increased dietary riboflavin.

5

Drugs Affecting the Cardiovascular System and the Blood

VI. **Antilipemic agents**
   A. Cholesterol-lowering agents
   B. Triglyceride-lowering agents
   C. Nursing diagnoses
   D. Nursing implementation factors
   E. Nursing evaluations

VII. **Anticoagulants**
   A. Heparin
   B. Oral anticoagulants
   C. Antiplatelet agents
   D. Nursing diagnoses
   E. Nursing implementation factors
   F. Nursing evaluations

VIII. **Thrombolytic agents**
   A. Examples
   B. Use/mechanism of action

   C. Adverse effects
   D. Contraindications
   E. Precautions
   F. Drug interactions
   G. Nursing diagnoses
   H. Nursing implementation factors
   I. Nursing evaluations

IX. **Hematinic agents**
   A. Iron
   B. Vitamin B_{12}
   C. Folic acid
   D. Erythropoietin
   E. Nursing diagnoses
   F. Nursing implementation factors
   G. Nursing evaluations

NURSING HIGHLIGHTS

1. The nurse should stress to clients the importance of nonmedical steps to reduce blood pressure: sodium restriction, alcohol restriction, aerobic exercise, good nutrition, weight loss, and stress reduction.
2. Similarly, the nurse should emphasize the importance of appropriate diet, exercise, and weight reduction to clients receiving antilipemic therapy.
3. In clients receiving long-term or lifelong medication, achieving compliance should be a major goal.
4. The nurse can encourage client compliance by periodically asking questions about the drug regimen, stressing the necessity of the medication, and cautioning client never to stop taking medication because he/she is feeling better.

GLOSSARY

angioedema—a vascular reaction of deep dermal, subcutaneous, or submucosal tissues characterized by localized edema and giant wheals
chronotropic—refers to heart rate
dromotropic—refers to impulse conduction
epistaxis—bleeding from the nose
hypertrichosis—excessive hair growth
inotropic—refers to strength of myocardial contractions
macrocytic (megaloblastic) anemia—a form of anemia marked by abnormally large red cells

microcytic anemia—a form of anemia marked by abnormally small red cells

pheochromocytoma—a tumor of the adrenal medulla or sympathetic para-ganglia whose most important symptom is hypertension

ENHANCED OUTLINE

I. Cardiac glycosides and inotropic agents

See text pages
_____

A. Cardiac glycosides
1. Examples: digoxin (Lanoxin), digitoxin (Crystodigin)
2. Use/mechanism of action: treat congestive heart failure and supraventricular arrhythmias by exerting positive inotropic effect, negative chronotropic and dromotropic effects
3. Adverse effects: anorexia, nausea, vomiting, diarrhea, abdominal pain, headache, confusion, skin rash, visual changes (flickering lights and snowflakes), dysrhythmias (see Nurse Alert, "Digitalis Toxicity")
4. Contraindications: acute myocardial infarction
5. Precautions: renal failure, severe pulmonary disease, hypothyroidism
6. Drug interactions
   a) Corticosteroids: hypokalemia
   b) Antacids: increased glycoside absorption
   c) Antiarrhythmic agents, cocaine, succinylcholine, sympathomimetics: increased risk of arrhythmias
   d) Calcium channel blockers: bradycardia
   e) Quinidine: increased glycoside serum level
   f) Spironolactone: increased glycoside half-life

B. Inotropic agents
1. Examples: amrinone (Inocor)
2. Use/mechanism of action: treat congestive heart failure by exerting positive inotropic effect and causing vasodilation
3. Adverse effects: nausea, vomiting, abdominal pain, arrhythmias, hypotension, thrombocytopenia, fever

! NURSE *ALERT* !

Digitalis Toxicity

Observe and question clients, especially the very young and the very old, for early signs of digitalis toxicity: visual changes, difficulty reading, and GI complaints, including nausea, vomiting, anorexia, and diarrhea.

4. Contraindications: bisulfite hypersensitivity
5. Precautions: severe valvular stenosis, pregnancy, lactation
6. Drug interactions: possible severe hypotension

C. Nursing diagnoses
1. Impaired adjustment to changed lifestyle
2. Hyperthermia related to hypersensitivity reaction to cardiac glycoside or amrinone
3. Activity intolerance related to adverse effect or poor effect of cardiac glycoside

D. Nursing implementation factors
1. Administration procedures
   a) Take apical pulse before administering each cardiac glycoside dose; do not administer if pulse is less than 60.
   b) Monitor blood pressure and heart rate during amrinone infusion.
2. Daily monitoring and measurements
   a) Monitor serum levels of potassium, creatinine, and digitalis.
   b) Monitor client's blood urea nitrogen (BUN).
   c) Check client's vital signs.
   d) Measure client's fluid intake and output and weight.
   e) Monitor white blood cell count (WBC) during amrinone therapy.
3. Points for client teaching
   a) Teach client to take pulse.
   b) Ensure that client is familiar with symptoms that should be reported immediately, especially sudden weight gain, edema, shortness of breath, nausea and vomiting, and visual disturbances.
   c) Advise client to prevent deterioration of inotropic agents by always storing medication in a tightly fitting, light- and moisture-resistant container.
   d) Instruct client to check with physician before taking any nonprescription drug, such as an antacid.

E. Nursing evaluations
1. Heart and respiratory rate are within normal limits, without rales or signs and symptoms of congestive heart failure.
2. Client is adapting well to altered lifestyle.
3. Client experiences improved activity tolerance.

II. Antianginals

A. Nitrates

See text pages

1. Examples: erythrityl tetranitrate (Cardilate); isosorbide dinitrate (Isordil, Sorbitrate); nitroglycerin (Deponit NTG Film, Nitrostat, Nitrogard); pentaerythritol tetranitrate (Peritrate, Duotrate)
2. Use/mechanism of action: treat angina by producing vasodilation through action on vascular smooth muscle
3. Adverse effects: orthostatic hypotension, dizziness, weakness, nausea, vomiting, headache, tolerance; cardiovascular collapse (rare)

   4. Contraindications: known hypersensitivity
   5. Precautions: dehydration, low systolic blood pressure, pregnancy, lactation
   6. Drug interactions
      a) Alcohol: severe hypotension
      b) Anticholinergics: delayed sublingual absorption due to dry mouth

B. Beta-blockers
   1. Examples: atenolol (Tenormin), metoprolol tartrate (Lopressor), nadolol (Corgard), propranolol (Inderal)
   2. Use/mechanism of action: treat angina by reducing myocardial oxygen demands through slowing of heart rate and decreasing force of contractions
   3. Adverse effects
      a) Cardiovascular: arrhythmias, orthostatic hypotension, bradycardia, congestive heart failure, edema, cold extremities
      b) Central nervous system (CNS): fatigue, vivid dreams, depression, insomnia, vertigo
      c) Gastrointestinal (GI): nausea, vomiting, diarrhea, constipation
      d) Respiratory: bronchospasm, dyspnea
      e) Skin: rash, pruritus
      f) Hematologic: hyperglycemia, hypoglycemia
   4. Contraindications: congestive heart failure, sinus bradycardia, heart block, cardiogenic shock, bronchospastic disease
   5. Precautions: diabetes, hypoglycemia, hepatic or renal impairment, respiratory disease
   6. Drug interactions: See Chapter 3, section VI,B,6.

C. Calcium channel blockers
   1. Examples: diltiazem (Cardizem); nicardipine (Cardene); nifedipine (Procardia); verapamil (Calan, Isoptin)
   2. Use/mechanism of action: treat angina by reducing myocardial oxygen demands by decreasing force of contractions and decreasing afterload
   3. Adverse effects: dizziness, headache, tachycardia, nausea, ankle edema, flushing
   4. Contraindications: severe hypotension
   5. Precautions: severe aortic stenosis, bradycardia, heart failure, cardiogenic shock, orthostatic hypotension, pregnancy
   6. Drug interactions
      a) Alcohol, other antihypertensives: increased hypotension
      b) Beta-blockers: bradycardia, hypotension, heart failure
      c) Carbamazepine, cyclosporine, quinidine, theophylline, cardiac glycosides: increased serum levels of these agents

        d) Disopyramide with diltiazem or verapamil: negative inotropic effects, sometimes fatal

D. Nursing diagnoses
  1. Anxiety related to medical condition
  2. Potential for injury related to hypotension
  3. Activity intolerance related to hypotension
  4. Pain related to unrelieved angina

E. Nursing implementation factors
  1. Administration procedures
    a) Place nitroglycerin sustained-release tablets between client's upper gum and lips.
    b) Have client lie or sit down while first dose is administered; check pulse and blood pressure before administering second nitrate dose.
    c) Choose a new site for subsequent doses when administering nitroglycerin ointment to minimize skin irritation.
    d) Avoid administering a beta-blocker or calcium channel blocker for acute angina attacks.
  2. Daily monitoring and measurements
    a) Take client's vital signs frequently; note decreases of pulse and heart rate or irregular rhythm.
    b) Monitor client for signs of hypotension, including systolic blood pressure less than 90 mm Hg, syncope, dizziness, weakness, clammy skin, nausea, vomiting, and tachycardia of more than 150 beats per minute.
    c) Monitor client for peripheral edema when beta-blockers and calcium channel blockers are being administered.
    d) Auscultate lungs frequently for signs of bronchoconstriction in client taking beta-blocker.
  3. Points for client teaching
    a) Tell client to go to emergency room of nearest hospital if angina is not relieved after taking three nitrate tablets at 5-minute intervals while resting.
    b) Tell client to take nitrate between meals for better absorption.
    c) Warn client not to stop taking nitrate abruptly because of risk of vasospasm.
    d) Caution client not to discontinue a beta-blocker abruptly because of risk of hypertension, arrhythmias, and acute myocardial infarction.
    e) Advise client on beta-blocker to notify physician if dyspnea, wheezing, or ankle edema occurs.

F. Nursing evaluations
  1. Client reports pain relief and decreased frequency of anginal attack.
  2. Client achieves improved activity tolerance.
  3. Client maintains normal body fluid balance with no edema.

I. Cardiac glycosides and inotropic agents	II. Antianginals	III. Antiarrhythmics	IV. Antihypertensives	V. Diuretics

See text pages
_____

III. Antiarrhythmics

A. Class I
   1. Example: moricizine (Ethmozine)
   2. Use/mechanism of action: treat cardiac electrical activity abnormalities by blocking sodium channels and slowing electrical conduction
   3. Adverse effects: proarrhythmias
   4. Contraindications: second- or third-degree atrioventricular (AV) block, cardiogenic shock, lactation, known hypersensitivity
   5. Precautions: severe hepatic or renal impairment, sick sinus syndrome, congestive heart failure
   6. Drug interactions
      a) Cimetidine: increased serum moricizine levels
      b) Theophylline: decreased theophylline half-life

B. Class IA
   1. Examples: disopyramide (Norpace), procainamide (Procan), quinidine (Cin-Quin)
   2. Use/mechanism of action: treat cardiac electrical activity abnormalities by blocking sodium channels and slowing electrical conduction
   3. Adverse effects: dry mouth, diarrhea, anorexia, GI distress, flushing, rash, urine retention
   4. Contraindications: digitalis intoxication with severe intraventricular conduction disorder, ectopic impulses, myasthenia gravis, known hypersensitivity
   5. Precautions: renal or hepatic impairment, pregnancy, lactation
   6. Drug interactions
      a) Disopyramide and anticholinergic: additive anticholinergic effects
      b) Disopyramide and verapamil: myocardial depression
      c) Procainamide and cimetidine or amiodarone: increased serum procainamide levels
      d) Quinidine and neuromuscular blockers: increased skeletal muscle relaxation
      e) Quinidine and oral anticoagulants: hypoprothrombinemia
      f) Quinidine and digoxin: increased serum digoxin levels, lessening efficacy of antiarrhythmic
      g) Quinidine and urine alkalinizers, cimetidine, or amiodarone: increased serum quinidine levels
      h) Quinidine or disopyramide with rifampin, phenytoin, or phenobarbital: increased antidysrrhythmic metabolism

C. Class IB
   1. Examples: lidocaine (Xylocaine), mexiletine (Mexitil), tocainide (Tonocard)

2. Use/mechanism of action: treat cardiac electrical activity abnormalities by decreasing action and potential duration and prolonging effective refractory period
3. Adverse effects: dizziness, anorexia, nausea, vomiting, tremors, chest pain
4. Contraindications: Stokes-Adams syndrome, Wolff-Parkinson-White syndrome, heart block, known hypersensitivity
5. Precautions: hypovolemia, severe congestive heart failure, shock, malignant hyperthermia
6. Drug interactions
   a) Other antiarrhythmics: additive or antagonistic effects
   b) Lidocaine with propranolol or cimetidine: induced lidocaine toxicity
   c) Mexiletine and rifampin or phenytoin: decreased mexiletine levels

D. Class IC
1. Examples: encainide (Enkaid), flecainide (Tambocor), indecainide (Decabid), propafenone (Rythmol)
2. Use/mechanism of action: treat cardiac electrical activity abnormalities by blocking sodium channels, depressing automaticity, and slowing spontaneous depolarization
3. Adverse effects: blurred vision, dizziness, headaches, constipation, nausea, chest pain
4. Contraindications: second- or third-degree AV block, lactation, known hypersensitivity
5. Precautions: sick sinus syndrome; congestive heart failure; myocardial dysfunction; prolonged P–R, QRS, or Q–T intervals; pacemaker previously implanted; pregnancy
6. Drug interactions
   a) Encainide and cimetidine: decreased encainide metabolism
   b) Encainide and other antiarrhythmics, beta-blockers, verapamil, diltiazem: additive effects on electrical conduction
   c) Flecainide or propafenone and digoxin: increased serum digoxin levels
   d) Flecainide and alkalinizing agents, cimetidine, propranolol: increased serum flecainide levels
   e) Flecainide and disopyramide, verapamil, diltiazem, beta-blockers: additive negative inotropic effects
   f) Indecainide and other antiarrhythmics: increased serum indecainide levels
   g) Propafenone and warfarin: increased prothrombin time
   h) Propafenone and metoprolol or propranolol: increased serum levels of metoprolol or propranolol
   i) Propafenone and quinidine: decreased propafenone metabolism

E. Class II (beta-blockers)
1. Examples: acebutolol (Sectral), esmolol (Brevibloc), propranolol (Inderal)
2. Use/mechanism of action: treat cardiac electrical activity abnormalities by blocking beta-receptors and decreasing sympathetic activity at sinoatrial and atrioventricular nodes, prolonging refractory period
3. Adverse effects: same as section VI,B,3 of Chapter 3

I. Cardiac glycosides and inotropic agents	II. Antianginals	III. Antiarrhythmics	IV. Antihypertensives	V. Diuretics

4. Contraindications: cardiogenic shock, sinus bradycardia, greater than first-degree heart block, bronchial asthma, congestive heart failure, known hypersensitivity
5. Precautions: bronchospasms, diabetes, hepatic or renal impairment, lactation, pregnancy
6. Drug interactions
   a) Phenothiazines: increased hypotension
   b) Sympathomimetics: decreased effectiveness of sympathomimetics
   c) Anticholinergics: hypertension, decreased effectiveness of antiarrhythmic
   d) Antihypertensives: increased hypotension
   e) Neuromuscular blockers: increased skeletal muscle relaxation
   f) Verapamil: increased cardiac depression
   g) Esmolol and digoxin: increased serum digoxin levels
   h) Esmolol and morphine: increased serum esmolol levels
   i) Propranolol and cimetidine: decreased propranolol metabolism, increasing risk of toxicity

F. Class III
   1. Examples: amiodarone (Cordarone), bretylium (Bretylol)
   2. Use/mechanism of action: treat cardiac electrical activity abnormalities by prolonging action potential
   3. Adverse effects: anorexia, headache, nausea, vomiting, constipation
   4. Contraindications: severe sinus node dysfunction, bradycardia with syncope, lactation
   5. Precautions: pregnancy
   6. Drug interactions
      a) Antihypertensives: profound hypotension
      b) Amiodarone and warfarin: increased hypoprothrombinemia
      c) Amiodarone and digoxin: increased serum digoxin levels
      d) Amiodarone and procainamide, quinidine, or phenytoin: increased amiodarone levels

G. Class IV (calcium channel blockers)
   1. Examples: diltiazem (Cardizem); verapamil (Calan, Isoptin); nicardipine (Cardene); nifedipine (Procardia)
   2. Use/mechanism of action: treat arrhythmias by decreasing force of myocardial contraction by blocking flow of calcium ions through cell membrane
   3. Adverse effects: dizziness, headache, tachycardia, nausea, ankle edema, flushing
   4. Contraindications: severe hypotension, cardiogenic shock, second- or third-degree AV block, sick sinus syndrome, severe congestive heart failure, Wolff-Parkinson-White syndrome, known hypersensitivity

5. Precautions: renal or hepatic impairment, lactation, pregnancy, severe aortic stenosis, bradycardia, heart failure, cardiogenic shock, orthostatic hypotension
6. Drug interactions
    a) Other antiarrhythmics: additive effects
    b) Antihypertensives: hypotension and heart failure
    c) Digoxin: digitalis toxicity

H. Other agents
  1. Examples: adenosine (Adenocard)
  2. Use/mechanism of action: treat cardiac electrical activity abnormalities by slowing conduction in atrioventricular node
  3. Adverse effects: facial flushing, dyspnea
  4. Contraindications: second- or third-degree AV block, sick sinus syndrome, atrial flutter, atrial fibrillation, ventricular tachycardia
  5. Precautions: asthma, pregnancy
  6. Drug interactions
    a) Carbamazepine: additive cardiovascular effects
    b) Dipyridamole: potentiation of adenosine effects
    c) Methylxanthines: adenosine antagonism

I. Nursing diagnoses
  1. Constipation related to anticholinergic effects
  2. Potential for injury related to arrhythmia
  3. Fatigue related to adverse CNS effects
  4. Activity intolerance related to arrhythmia

J. Nursing implementation factors
  1. Administration procedures
    a) Refrain from administering a class I drug with food unless prescribed.
    b) Do not use solutions containing epinephrine when lidocaine is prescribed to treat arrhythmias.
    c) Administer mexiletine and tocainide with food to minimize GI distress.
  2. Daily monitoring and measurements
    a) Watch for signs of congestive heart failure, such as hypotension, peripheral edema, irregular heartbeat, shortness of breath, crackles, and jugular vein distention.
    b) Monitor electrolyte levels.
    c) Monitor serum drug levels.
    d) Watch for signs of lidocaine toxicity, such as confusion or restlessness.
  3. Points for client teaching
    a) Tell female client to notify physician if she plans to become pregnant or becomes pregnant during antiarrhythmic therapy.
    b) Have clients weigh themselves daily and report a gain or loss of more than 2 lb per day.
    c) Teach clients the signs of hypokalemia and congestive heart disease.
    d) Teach clients how to take a pulse.

K. Nursing evaluations
1. Client's heart rate is within normal limits.
2. Client achieves acceptable arrhythmia control, as determined by physician.

IV. Antihypertensives

See text pages
_____

A. Central adrenergic inhibitors
1. Examples: clonidine (Catapres), methyldopa (Aldomet), guanabenz (Wytensin), guanfacine (Tenex)
2. Use/mechanism of action: treat hypertension by inhibiting vasoconstriction by stimulating cardiovascular center of brain, decreasing outflow of sympathetic vasoconstrictor impulses
3. Adverse effects: itching, rashes, urticaria, hypotension, bradycardia, congestive heart failure, fever, dizziness, syncope, libido changes, dry mouth, edema, impotence
4. Contraindications: pregnancy
5. Precautions: cerebrovascular disease, coronary insufficiency, diabetes, chronic renal failure, recent myocardial infarction, mental depression
6. Drug interactions
    a) Beta-blockers: paradoxical hypertension
    b) CNS depressants: enhance CNS depression of clonidine
    c) Tricyclic antidepressants and MAO (monoamine oxidase) inhibitors: decreased antihypertensive effect

B. Alpha-adrenergic blockers
1. Examples: phenoxybenzamine (Dibenzyline), phentolamine (Regitine), ergotamine tartrate (Ergomar)
2. Use/mechanism of action: treat hypertension by inhibiting action of alpha-receptors in vascular smooth muscle, causing vasodilation
3. Adverse effects
    a) Cardiovascular: orthostatic hypotension, bradycardia, tachycardia, edema, dyspnea, angina, myocardial infarction, cerebrovascular spasm
    b) CNS: paresthesias, muscle weakness, fatigue, depression, insomnia, lethargy, sedation, vertigo, syncope, confusion, headache
    c) Ear, nose, throat: nasal congestion, tinnitus, dry mouth
    d) GI: nausea, vomiting, heartburn, diarrhea, cramping, exacerbated peptic ulcers
    e) Genitourinary: urinary frequency, incontinence, impotence, priapism
4. Contraindications: myocardial infarction, coronary insufficiency, angina
5. Precautions: pregnancy, lactation

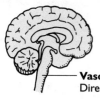

Vasomotor center of brain
Directly affected by central adrenergic inhibitors

Sympathetic ganglion
Control center

Blood vessel
Directly affected by peripheral adrenergic inhibitors, arteriolar dilators, and arteriolar and venous dilators

Heart
Carotid and aortic sinuses provide feedback to vasomotor center

Kidneys
Directly affected by diuretics, which decrease sodium, thereby decreasing blood vessel constriction

Figure 5–1
Effects of Drugs on Physiologic Processes Related to Hypertension

   6. Drug interactions
       a) Ergotamine and nitroglycerine: excessive vasodilation and increased ergot availability
       b) Other hypertensives: potentiation of hypotensive effects

C. Beta-adrenergic blockers
   1. Examples: propranolol (Inderal), metoprolol (Lopressor), nadolol (Corgard), timolol (Blocadren)
   2. Use/mechanism of action: treat hypertension by competing with epinephrine to occupy beta-adrenergic receptors in heart (beta$_1$) and/or peripheral circulation, pulmonary airways, and CNS (beta$_2$)
   3. Adverse effects
       a) Cardiovascular: arrhythmias, orthostatic hypotension, bradycardia, congestive heart failure, edema, cold extremities
       b) CNS: fatigue, vivid dreams, depression, insomnia, vertigo
       c) GI: nausea, vomiting, diarrhea, constipation
       d) Respiratory: bronchospasm, dyspnea
       e) Skin: rash, pruritus
       f) Hematologic: hyperglycemia, hypoglycemia
   4. Contraindications: congestive heart failure, sinus bradycardia, heart block, cardiogenic shock, bronchospastic disease
   5. Precautions: diabetes, hypoglycemia, hepatic or renal impairment, respiratory disease
   6. Drug interactions (see Chapter 3, section VI,B,6)

D. Ganglionic blockers
   1. Examples: mecamylamine (Inversine), trimethaphan camsylate (Arfonad), hexamethonium

2. Use/mechanism of action: treat hypertension by competing with acetylcholine to occupy cholinergic receptors in autonomic ganglia, preventing vasoconstriction
3. Adverse effects: tachycardia, bradycardia, orthostatic hypotension, restlessness, weakness, sedation, cycloplegia, mydriasis, nausea, vomiting, anorexia, loss of GI tract tone, respiratory depression
4. Contraindications: anemia, hypovolemia, shock, asphyxia, respiratory insufficiency
5. Precautions: allergies, debilitation, advanced age
6. Drug interactions
   a) Anesthetics: increased hypotension
   b) Muscle relaxants: increased neuromuscular blockade and prolonged respiratory depression

E. Calcium channel blockers
   1. Examples: diltiazem (Cardizem); nicardipine (Cardene); nifedipine (Procardia); verapamil (Calan, Isoptin)
   2. Use/mechanism of action: reduce hypertension and treat Raynaud's phenomenon (nicardipine and nifedipine) by decreasing force of myocardial contraction by blocking flow of calcium ions through cell membrane
   3. Adverse effects: dizziness, headache, tachycardia, nausea, ankle edema, flushing
   4. Contraindications: severe hypotension
   5. Precautions: severe aortic stenosis, bradycardia, heart failure, cardiogenic shock, orthostatic hypotension, pregnancy
   6. Drug interactions
      a) Alcohol, other antihypertensives: increased hypotension
      b) Beta-blockers: bradycardia, hypotension, heart failure
      c) Carbamazepine, cyclosporine, quinidine, theophylline, cardiac glycosides: increased serum levels of these agents
      d) Disopyramide with diltiazem or verapamil: negative inotropic effects, sometimes fatal

F. Peripheral adrenergic inhibitors
   1. Examples: guanadrel sulfate (Hylorel), guanethidine monosulfate (Ismelin), reserpine (Serpasil)
   2. Use/mechanism of action: treat hypertension by reducing vascular wall tone through reduction of sympathetic nervous system stimulation of blood vessels
   3. Adverse effects: itching, rashes, urticaria, hypotension, bradycardia, congestive heart failure, fever, dizziness, syncope, libido changes, dry mouth, edema, impotence
   4. Contraindications: congestive heart failure, pheochromocytoma

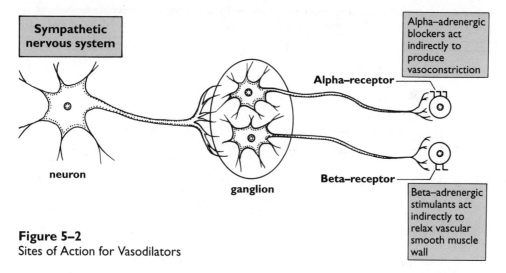

Figure 5–2
Sites of Action for Vasodilators

5. Precautions: advanced age, pregnancy, cerebrovascular and peripheral vascular disease, febrile states, renal and hepatic impairment, asthma
6. Drug interactions
   a) Diuretics: increase in hypotensive effects
   b) Potassium-sparing diuretics: hypokalemia
   c) MAO inhibitors: severe hypertension

G. Vascular smooth muscle relaxants (vasodilators)
   1. Examples: diazoxide (Hyperstat IV); hydralazine (Apresoline); minoxidil (Loniten); sodium nitroprusside (Nipride, Nitropress)
   2. Use/mechanism of action: treat hypertension by relaxing smooth muscle in blood vessel walls to cause peripheral vasodilation
   3. Adverse effects: diarrhea, nausea, vomiting, anorexia, tachycardia, headache, edema, flushing, ankle edema; unusual hair growth (minoxidil)
   4. Contraindications
      a) Diazoxide: compensatory hypertension
      b) Hydralazine: coronary artery disease, rheumatic mitral valvular disease, myocardial infarction, tachycardia, lupus erythematosus
      c) Minoxidil: pheochromocytoma
      d) Sodium nitroprusside: impaired cerebral circulation, compensatory hypertension
   5. Precautions
      a) Diazoxide: thiazide or sulfonamide hypersensitivity, impaired cerebral or cardiac circulation
      b) Hydralazine: coronary artery disease, rheumatic mitral valvular disease, renal impairment
      c) Minoxidil: recent myocardial infarction, renal impairment
      d) Sodium nitroprusside: renal or hepatic impairment, vitamin B_{12} deficiency
   6. Drug interactions
      a) Anticoagulants and diazoxide: increased anticoagulant effects
      b) Minoxidil and guanethidine: increased hypotension

      c) Minoxidil with diazoxide, nitrates, or nitroprusside: severe hypotension

  H. ACE (angiotensin-converting enzyme) inhibitors

    1. Examples: captopril (Capoten); enalapril (Vasotec); lisinopril (Prinivil, Zestril)

    2. Use/mechanism of action: reduce blood pressure by blocking conversion of angiotensin I to angiotensin II, a powerful vasoconstrictor

    3. Adverse effects: headache, dizziness, fatigue, GI distress, neutropenia, agranulocytosis, rash, proteinuria

    4. Contraindications: pregnancy

    5. Precautions: impaired renal function, valvular stenosis, lactation

    6. Drug interactions

      a) Other hypertensives: increased hypotension

      b) Nonsteroidal anti-inflammatory drugs (NSAIDs): decreased response when NSAIDs are concurrently administered

 I. Nursing diagnoses

    1. Anxiety related to medical condition

    2. Fluid volume excess related to dependent edema

    3. Potential for injury related to orthostatic hypotension

 J. Nursing implementation factors

    1. Administration procedures

      a) All antihypertensives: Record blood pressure, pulse, and mental state before administering drug.

      b) Central adrenergic inhibitors: Ensure that baseline conjugated bile salts (CBS), electrolyte, creatinine, BUN, and liver function tests have been completed before first administration of drug.

      c) Alpha-adrenergic blockers: Administer oral drugs with milk to minimize GI effects.

      d) Beta-adrenergic blockers

        (1) Administer oral drug before meals or at bedtime to speed absorption.

        (2) Administer any needed antacids several hours before or after beta-blocker administration.

        (3) Check client's apical pulse rate before drug administration; if under 60, inform physician before proceeding.

      e) Ganglionic blockers

        (1) Give smaller doses in morning, when response is generally greater.

        (2) Administer trimethaphan by continuous infusion without mixing another drug in syringe; discontinue IV slowly.

        (3) Administer trimethaphan when client is supine or seated in head-down position.

f) Calcium channel blockers
   (1) Administer calcium channel blocker between meals to enhance absorption.
   (2) Take client's pulse before each dose; withhold drug if pulse is below 60.
   (3) Check blood pressure and withhold drug if systolic pressure is less than 90 (see Client Teaching Checklist, "Calcium Channel Blockers").
g) Vascular smooth muscle relaxants
   (1) Do not combine other drugs in same syringe with sodium nitroprusside; avoid extravasation.
   (2) Administer sodium nitroprusside using a microdrip regulator or automatic infusion pump.
h) ACE inhibitors
   (1) Monitor for hypotension during initial administration if client is also taking another antihypertensive drug.
   (2) Administer captopril between meals.

2. Daily monitoring and measurements
   a) All hypertensives
      (1) Take blood pressure and pulse.
      (2) Note any change in blood pressure when client rises from supine position.
   b) Central adrenergic inhibitors
      (1) Monitor client for dizziness, confusion, visual changes, bradycardia, hypotension, or depression; in case of occurrence, withhold drug and report to physician.
      (2) Monitor weight and fluid intake and output daily; report any significant weight increase.
   c) Alpha-adrenergic blockers
      (1) Note symptoms of light-headedness, weakness, or altered mental functioning; elevate client's bed side rails and give assistance if CNS symptoms occur.

✔ CLIENT TEACHING CHECKLIST ✔

Calcium Channel Blockers

Explanations to the client who is taking calcium channel blockers:

✔ If you are taking nitroglycerin concurrently for acute angina, keep a journal of anginal episodes and report any changes that occur with calcium channel blocker therapy.

✔ Stand up slowly to minimize orthostatic hypotension.

✔ You will be taught how to take your pulse; report a heart rate under 60.

✔ Take a missed dose as soon as possible unless it is time for the next dose, in which case you should skip the missed dose.

✔ It is very important that you keep follow-up appointments.

(2) Monitor client taking ergotamine for signs of vascular insufficiency, including numbness, coldness, tingling, or weakness in extremities.

(3) Notify physician immediately if client reports chest pain.

d) Beta-adrenergic blockers

(1) Monitor vital signs, fluid intake and output, breath sounds, and peripheral circulation before and during drug administration.

(2) Monitor blood glucose levels in clients with diabetes.

(3) Use safety precautions, including use of bed side rails, if client develops adverse CNS effects.

e) Ganglionic blockers

(1) Closely monitor clients with histories of allergies.

(2) Watch for nutritional deficits or weight loss.

(3) Monitor client for rebound hypertension during drug withdrawal.

f) Calcium channel blockers

(1) Check electrocardiogram for prolonged P–R interval.

(2) Monitor client for signs of congestive heart failure.

g) Peripheral adrenergic inhibitors

(1) Monitor for dizziness, confusion, bradycardia, diarrhea, and hypotension; withhold drug and report symptoms if they occur.

(2) Supervise client's ambulation until response to drug has been established.

h) Vascular smooth muscle relaxants

(1) Measure body weight, fluid intake, and output.

(2) Check results of complete blood count (CBC), antinuclear antibody titer test, and lupus erythematosus cell preparation tests before initiating hydralazine therapy and periodically thereafter.

(3) Monitor serum electrolytes with diazoxide and minoxidil.

i) ACE inhibitors

(1) Check blood pressure and heart rate.

(2) Monitor periodically for proteinuria.

(3) Take WBC count.

(4) Monitor serum BUN, creatinine, and potassium.

(5) Measure fluid intake and output and daily weight.

(6) Monitor for signs of angioedema.

3. Points for client teaching (see Client Teaching Checklist, "Points to Cover about Antihypertensives")

a) Advise client not to drive or operate dangerous machinery until effects of medication have been established.

b) Caution client that drinking alcohol may cause excessive drowsiness.

Points to Cover about Antihypertensives

Emphasize the following points to a client beginning antihypertensive therapy:

✔ Antihypertensive therapy is usually administered on a long-term basis, possibly for life.
✔ Follow-up visits to monitor drug levels and blood pressure are very important.
✔ Never discontinue medication simply because you are feeling better.
✔ Monitor pulse and blood pressure; you will be taught to do this.
✔ Change position slowly to avoid dizziness.
✔ You will be taught to recognize the symptoms of hypertensive crisis brought on by missed doses, including anxiety, sweating, tachycardia, insomnia, salivation, muscle pain, and stomach pain.
✔ Report serious adverse effects immediately without discontinuing drug.
✔ Be aware that sexual problems may occur but that they are not a cause for alarm, because changes in drug or dosage will usually resolve them.
✔ Be aware that holistic measures (weight control, diet, exercise, stress reduction) enhance the effect of antihypertensives.

    c) Tell client to avoid OTC medications that contain alcohol unless physician has approved them.
    d) Show client methods for minimizing the effects of orthostatic hypotension, dizziness, and light-headedness.
    e) Encourage client to monitor weight.
    f) Teach client to monitor pulse and blood pressure.
    g) Tell client that medication must be continued even if he/she feels well.
    h) Emphasize that client should report hypertension, hypotension, syncope, persistent dizziness, or chest pain.
    i) Advise client to reduce salt intake.

K. Nursing evaluations
    1. Client's blood pressure is within normal range.
    2. Client monitors own pulse, blood pressure, and weight.
    3. Client is alert to the possibility of orthostatic hypotension.
    4. Client knows which symptoms to report.

V. Diuretics

A. Thiazide diuretics

    1. Examples: chlorothiazide (Diuril); chlorthalidone (Hygroton); hydrochlorothiazide (HydroDIURIL, Esidrex, Oretic); indapamide (Lozol); metolazone (Diulo, Zaroxolyn)
    2. Use/mechanism of action: treat edema, congestive heart failure, hypertension by increasing water and sodium excretion through inhibition of sodium reabsorption in distal tubule of kidney

> See text pages

      3. Adverse effects: blood volume depletion, orthostatic hypotension, hyponatremia, hypokalemia, hypercalcemia, hypophosphatemia

      4. Contraindications: sulfonamide hypersensitivity, severe renal or hepatic impairment; lactation

      5. Precautions: renal or hepatic impairment, progressive liver disease, pregnancy

      6. Drug interactions

         a) Lithium: toxicity due to reduced excretion

         b) NSAIDs: reduced effectiveness of diuretic

         c) Cardiac glycosides: digitalis toxicity

         d) Insulin: hyponatremia, thiazide resistance, hyperglycemia

  B. Loop diuretics

      1. Examples: bumetanide (Bumex), ethacrynate (Edecrin), furosemide (Lasix)

      2. Use/mechanism of action: treat edema and congestive heart failure by increasing urinary volume by inhibiting sodium and chloride reabsorption in loop of Henle and distal tubule of kidney

      3. Adverse effects: blood volume depletion, orthostatic hypotension, hyponatremia, hypokalemia, hypercalcemia, hypophosphatemia

      4. Contraindications: hypersensitivity, anuria, pregnancy, lactation

      5. Precautions: renal dysfunction

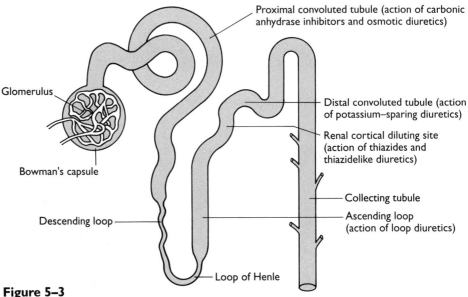

Figure 5–3
Sites of Diuretic Action in Nephron

6. Drug interactions
   a) Lithium: toxicity due to reduced excretion
   b) Aminoglycosides: ototoxicity
   c) Cisplatin: additive toxicity
   d) Cardiac glycosides: digitalis-induced arrhythmias
   e) NSAIDs: reduced effectiveness of diuretic

C. Potassium-sparing diuretics
   1. Examples: amiloride (Midamor), spironolactone (Aldactone), triamterene (Dyrenium)
   2. Use/mechanism of action: treat edema and congestive heart failure by acting on distal tubule to increase excretion of sodium and bicarbonate, while conserving potassium
   3. Adverse effects: hyperkalemia, megaloblastic anemia, orthostatic hypotension, GI distress
   4. Contraindications: anuria, hypersensitivity, renal insufficiency, lactation
   5. Precautions: pregnancy
   6. Drug interactions
      a) Antihypertensives: additive hypotension
      b) Potassium supplements: hyperkalemia
      c) ACE inhibitors: hyperkalemia

D. Carbonic anhydrase diuretics
   1. Examples: acetazolamide (Diamox)
   2. Use/mechanism of action: treat edema and glaucoma by increasing urinary excretion of sodium, potassium, bicarbonate, and water and reducing intraocular pressure
   3. Adverse effects: paresthesias, hearing loss, anorexia, GI distress
   4. Contraindications: sulfonamide hypersensitivity, severe kidney or liver disease, acidosis; electrolyte imbalance with concurrent salicylates
   5. Precautions: pregnancy, lactation, diabetes
   6. Drug interactions: no significant drug interactions

E. Osmotic diuretics
   1. Examples: mannitol (Osmitrol); urea (Aquacara, Carbamide, Ureuert, Ureaphil)
   2. Use/mechanism of action: treat edema, congestive heart failure, and acute renal failure and reduce intracranial and intraocular pressure by increasing urination by increasing osmotic pressure of glomerular filtrate, inhibiting reabsorption of water and electrolytes
   3. Adverse effects: circulatory overload and tachycardia during infusion, electrolyte imbalances, volume depletion, cellular dehydration, headache, nausea, vomiting
   4. Contraindications: anuric renal disease, severe pulmonary congestion or edema, active intracranial bleeding, increased oliguria and azotemia
   5. Precautions: pregnancy
   6. Drug interactions: no significant drug interactions

F. Nursing diagnoses
  1. Altered urinary elimination related to diuretic agent
  2. Potential for injury related to postural hypotension
  3. Fluid volume deficit related to blood volume depletion
  4. Potential sleep pattern disturbance related to nocturnal diuresis

G. Nursing implementation factors
  1. Administration procedures
    a) Administer diuretic early in day to avoid nocturnal diuresis.
    b) Administer IV loop diuretic over 1–2 minutes to prevent adverse reactions.
  2. Daily monitoring and measurements
    a) Check weight daily for gain or loss of more than 2 lb per day.
    b) Assess client for signs of dehydration.
    c) Measure fluid input and output throughout therapy.
    d) Watch for signs and symptoms of electrolyte imbalance and glucose intolerance.
      (1) Hyponatremia: dizziness, weakness
      (2) Hyperglycemia: polyuria, polydipsia, polyphagia, weight loss
      (3) Hypokalemia: drowsiness, paresthesia, muscle cramps, hyporeflexia
      (4) Hyperkalemia: confusion, hyperexcitability, muscle weakness, flaccid paralysis, arrhythmias
    e) Monitor for signs of hypovolemia: tachycardia, hypotension, dyspnea
  3. Points for client teaching
    a) Warn female client to let physician know if she becomes pregnant or plans to become pregnant during diuretic therapy.
    b) Tell client that periodic blood tests will be necessary to evaluate imbalances that may occur during diuretic therapy.
    c) Teach client to recognize and report signs of hypokalemia.
    d) Tell client to rise slowly to minimize effects of orthostatic hypotension.
    e) Tell client to take diuretic early in day to avoid nocturia.
    f) Teach client taking a potassium-sparing diuretic to recognize signs of hyperkalemia.

H. Nursing evaluations
  1. Client's fluid intake and output are normal.
  2. Client's blood pressure is within normal range.
  3. Client's edema is decreased.
  4. Urinary output is increased.
  5. Intraocular pressure is decreased.

VI. Antilipemic agents

See text pages
_____

A. Cholesterol-lowering agents
   1. Examples: cholestyramine (Questran), colestipol (Colestid), lovastatin (Mevacor), probucol (Lorelco)
   2. Use/mechanism of action: treat hyperlipidemia by lowering circulating levels of low-density lipoproteins (LDL) or by interfering with cholesterol synthesis
   3. Adverse effects: abdominal pain, distention, constipation, flatulence, nausea, vomiting, diarrhea, headache, anorexia, weakness, fatigue
   4. Contraindications: complete biliary obstruction, liver disease, elevated serum transaminase, pregnancy, lactation
   5. Precautions: constipation, history of liver disease, high alcohol consumption
   6. Drug interactions
      a) Oral anticoagulants: increased risk of clotting
      b) Corticosteroids, acetaminophen, cardiac glycosides, iron preparations, thiazide-type diuretics: decreased GI tract absorption of these compounds, reducing their effectiveness
      c) Probucol and clofibrate: additive effects
      d) Lovastatin and immunosuppressant, gemfibrozil or niacin: increased risk of myopathy

B. Triglyceride-lowering agents
   1. Examples: gemfibrozil (Lopid), clofibrate (Atromid-S)
   2. Use/mechanism of action: treat hyperlipidemia by decreasing lipoprotein and triglyceride synthesis
   3. Adverse effects: increased incidence of cholelithiasis, hypersensitivity reactions
   4. Contraindications: hepatic or renal impairment, biliary cirrhosis, lactation, known hypersensitivity
   5. Precautions: pregnancy, peptic ulcer
   6. Drug interactions
      a) Oral anticoagulants: increased anticoagulant effects
      b) Sulfonylureas: increased hypoglycemia

C. Nursing diagnoses
   1. Altered nutrition, less than body requirements, related to adverse GI effects of antilipemic
   2. Constipation related to adverse GI effects of antilipemic
   3. Impaired physical mobility related to weakness caused by bile-sequestering agent
   4. Pain related to biliary colic from cholelithiasis caused by triglyceride-lowering agent

D. Nursing implementation factors
   1. Administration procedures
      a) Administer gemfibrozil in 2 daily divided doses 30 minutes before meals.
      b) Introduce and titrate bile-sequestering agent slowly to minimize adverse GI effects.

      2. Daily monitoring and measurements
        a) Assess client for constipation.
        b) Monitor liver function studies and WBC.
        c) Measure blood triglyceride and cholesterol levels.
        d) Evaluate serum creatine phosphokinase in clofibrate client.
        e) Monitor prothrombin times for client on concurrent oral anticoagulant therapy.
      3. Points for client teaching
        a) Encourage client to drink fluids, increase dietary fiber intake, and exercise daily to prevent constipation.
        b) Warn client to notify all physicians prescribing medication that he/she is receiving a bile-sequestering agent.
        c) Tell client to have cholesterol levels checked regularly.
        d) Explain the importance of liver function tests to client beginning to take lovastatin or triglyceride-lowering agent.

E. Nursing evaluations
    1. Client triglyceride and/or cholesterol levels are within normal range within 3 months.
    2. Client avoids constipation by increasing fluid and fiber intake.

VII. Anticoagulants

See text pages

A. Heparin
    1. Example: heparin
    2. Use/mechanism of action: reduce blood clotting by interfering with conversion of prothrombin to thrombin and fibrinogen to fibrin
    3. Adverse effects: bleeding, thrombocytopenia, hypersensitivity, alopecia with long-term therapy
    4. Contraindications: severe thrombocytopenia, uncontrolled bleeding site, known hypersensitivity
    5. Precautions: pregnancy, history of allergy or diseases with risk of hemorrhage
    6. Drug interactions
      a) Oral anticoagulants, antiplatelet agents: increased risk of bleeding
      b) Digitalis, quinidine, tetracycline, neomycin, penicillin, phenothiazines, antihistamines: inactivation of heparin if administered in same syringe
      c) Nicotine: possible inactivation of heparin
      d) Nitroglycerin: inhibition of heparin

B. Oral anticoagulants
    1. Examples: dicumarol (Dicumarol Pulvules), warfarin (Coumadin)
    2. Use/mechanism of action: reduce blood clotting by altering synthesis of vitamin K–dependent clotting factors such as prothrombin

3. Adverse effects: bleeding
4. Contraindications: pregnancy, tendency to hemorrhage, blood dyscrasias, recent CNS surgery, uncontrolled bleeding site
5. Precautions: lactation, hepatic or renal impairment, hypertension, severe diabetes, polycythemia vera
6. Drug interactions
   a) Salicylates, phenylbutazone, sulfinpyrazone, indomethacin, clofibrate, steroids, chloral hydrate, chloramphenicol, disulfiram, heparin, gemfibrozil, meclofenamate, mefenamic acid, metronidazole, miconazole, nalidixic acid, piroxicam, allopurinol, cimetidine, dextrothyroxine, erythromycin, glucagon, sulindac, thyroid hormones: increased risk of bleeding
   b) Phenytoin: increased risk of phenytoin toxicity
   c) Alcohol, vitamin K–rich foods: increased clotting

C. Antiplatelet agents
   1. Examples: aspirin, dipyridamole (Persantine), sulfinpyrazone (Anturane)
   2. Use/mechanism of action: reduce blood clotting by interfering with platelet activity
   3. Adverse effects: GI irritation (see Nurse Alert, "Aspirin and Salicylism")
   4. Contraindications: bleeding disorder
   5. Precautions: renal impairment, hypoprothrombinemia, vitamin K deficiency, thrombocytopenia, lactation
   6. Drug interactions
      a) Heparin, oral anticoagulants, dipyridamole: increased risk of bleeding with aspirin
      b) Sulfinpyrazone: antagonism of sulfinpyrazone's uricosuric effects when taken with aspirin
      c) Methotrexate, valproic acid: increased risk of toxicity when taken with aspirin

D. Nursing diagnoses
   1. Impaired tissue integrity related to gastric mucosa injury
   2. Potential for injury related to bleeding

E. Nursing implementation factors
   1. Administration procedures
      a) Monitor activated partial prothrombin time (APPT) throughout heparin infusion and partial prothrombin time (PPT) for warfarin.

! NURSE *ALERT* !

Aspirin and Salicylism

High doses of aspirin can cause salicylism, diagnosed by dizziness, tinnitus, difficulty hearing, nausea, vomiting, diarrhea, confusion, and lethargy.

        b) Administer aspirin or sulfinpyrazone with food or milk to minimize gastric irritation.

    2. Daily monitoring and measurements

        a) Monitor PPT or APPT and platelet count.

        b) Watch vital signs, hemoglobin level, and hematocrit for signs of bleeding.

        c) Check urine, stool, and emesis for occult bleeding.

        d) Watch for epistaxis, gingival bleeding, or ecchymoses.

        e) Check for signs of thrombophlebitis, including calf pain, tenderness, and redness.

    3. Points for client teaching

        a) Tell client to use electric razor and soft-bristle toothbrush to minimize bleeding.

        b) Caution client not to take any other prescription or OTC drugs without first checking with physician.

        c) Advise client to report any excessive bruising or blood in stool.

        d) Teach client on high doses of aspirin how to recognize signs and symptoms of salicylism.

        e) Caution client to advise dentist of drug regimen prior to any dental work.

F. Nursing evaluations

    1. APPT and/or PPT are within therapeutic range.

    2. Client takes aspirin with food to avoid gastric mucosa injury.

    3. Client shows no signs of obvious or occult bleeding.

VIII. Thrombolytic agents

See text pages
_____

A. Examples: alteplase (Activase); anistreplase (Eminase); streptokinase (Kabikinase, Streptase); urokinase (Abbokinase)

B. Use/mechanism of action: dissolve thrombi by converting plasminogen to plasmin, permitting the hydrolysis of clot fibrin

C. Adverse effects: bleeding, allergic responses

D. Contraindications: active internal bleeding, recent cerebrovascular accident, intracranial or intraspinal surgery, intracranial neoplasm, severe hypertension, known hypersensitivity

E. Precautions: recent major surgery or organ biopsy, recent trauma, hypertension, subacute bacterial endocarditis, hemostatic defects, diabetic hemorrhagic retinopathy

F. Drug interactions: increased risk of bleeding with heparin, oral anticoagulants, antiplatelet drugs, NSAIDs

G. Nursing diagnoses
   1. Anxiety related to medical condition
   2. Potential for injury related to bleeding

H. Nursing implementation factors
   1. Administration procedures
      a) Ask client to execute informed consent document.
      b) Conduct coagulation studies before and after administration.
      c) Monitor client for bleeding, paying special attention to puncture and wound sites.
      d) Monitor client for arrhythmias.
   2. Daily monitoring and measurements
      a) Observe for signs of microembolism, including skin mottling, pallor, or cyanosis.
      b) Do not administer IM injections or insert new arterial lines for 24 hours after thrombolytic agent administration.
      c) After intracoronary thrombolytic therapy, immobilize client's leg and leave femoral venous and arterial sheaths in place for 24 hours.
      d) Have antiarrhythmia and antihypersensitivity agents close at hand.
   3. Points for client teaching
      a) Encourage client and family to ask questions and express fears.
      b) Tell client to inform nurse of adverse reactions or worsening chest pain.

I. Nursing evaluations
   1. Clot is dissolved.
   2. Client experiences no bleeding or complications.

IX. Hematinic agents

See text pages
_____

A. Iron
   1. Example: iron
   2. Use/mechanism of action: treat anemia by reversing the iron deficiency that causes microcytic anemia
   3. Adverse effects: GI irritation; acute hypersensitivity to iron dextran
   4. Contraindications: primary hemochromatosis, acute infectious kidney disease, peptic ulcer, enteritis, ulcerative colitis, known hypersensitivity
   5. Precautions: severe liver impairment, asthma, pregnancy, lactation
   6. Drug interactions
      a) Tetracyclines, penicillamine, methyldopa: decreased absorption of these drugs
      b) Cholestyramine, colestipol: reduced serum iron levels
      c) Coffee, tea, eggs, milk: inhibition of iron absorption
      d) Vitamin E: impaired effectiveness of iron therapy in children

B. Vitamin B_{12}
   1. Example: vitamin B_{12}
   2. Use/mechanism of action: treat anemia by reversing vitamin B_{12} deficiencies that cause macrocytic (megaloblastic) anemia

3. Adverse effects: hypersensitivity responses to parenterally administered agent
4. Contraindications: early Leber's disease, known hypersensitivity
5. Precautions: history of gout
6. Drug interactions: inhibition of hematopoietic activity of vitamin B_{12} when administered with chloramphenicol

C. Folic acid
   1. Example: folic acid (Folvite)
   2. Use/mechanism of action: treat anemia by reversing folic acid deficiencies that cause macrocytic (megaloblastic) anemia
   3. Adverse effects: allergic responses
   4. Contraindications: anemia of unknown cause
   5. Precautions: pernicious anemia
   6. Drug interactions
      a) Anticonvulsants: possible interference with anticonvulsant effectiveness when folic acid is administered at high doses
      b) Glutethimide, isoniazid, cycloserine, oral contraceptives: inhibition of folic acid absorption

D. Erythropoietin (Epogen)
   1. Example: iron
   2. Use/mechanism of action: treat anemia by stimulating RBC production
   3. Adverse effects: hypertension, headache, arthralgias, nausea, edema, fatigue, diarrhea, chest pain
   4. Contraindications: uncontrolled hypertension, known albumin hypersensitivity
   5. Precautions: porphyria, pregnancy, lactation
   6. Drug interactions: decreased effectiveness of heparin when administered with erythropoietin, such as during hemodialysis

E. Nursing diagnoses
   1. Constipation related to adverse GI effects of iron supplementation
   2. Impaired tissue integrity related to inflammation at site of iron or erythropoietin administration
   3. Fatigue related to anemia

F. Nursing implementation factors
   1. Administration procedures
      a) Infuse iron dextran IV slowly, at a rate of 1 ml/minute.
      b) Administer iron dextran IM by Z-track technique to avoid leakage into subcutaneous tissue.
      c) Keep emergency equipment at hand in case of anaphylaxis related to iron dextran or vitamin B_{12} hypersensitivity.

2. Daily monitoring and measurements
   a) Measure serum iron level and CBC.
   b) Monitor client receiving iron dextran or parenteral vitamin B_{12} for hypersensitivity reaction.
   c) Check hematocrit and reticulocyte count in macrocytic anemia clients.
3. Points for client teaching
   a) Suggest diet changes appropriate for type of anemia.
   b) Explain to client that iron preparations normally darken the stool but that physician should be contacted if cramping or bloody stool occurs.
   c) Tell client how to prevent or relieve constipation.

G. Nursing evaluations
   1. Client has more energy and less shortness of breath.
   2. Client avoids constipation by increasing dietary fiber and fluid intake.
   3. Client has no irritation at injection site.

1. To detect early signs of digitalis toxicity, the nurse should make frequent assessments of the client's:
   a. Vision.
   b. Hearing.
   c. Urine output.
   d. Gait.

2. The client who is taking digoxin (Lanoxin) for congestive heart failure should be taught to increase dietary intake of:
   a. Sodium.
   b. Pyridoxine (vitamin B$_6$).
   c. Calcium.
   d. Potassium.

3. When sublingual nitroglycerin tablets are prescribed to relieve acute anginal pain, the client should be taught to:
   a. Store the tablets in the refrigerator.
   b. Take no more than 5 tablets per day.
   c. Go to the emergency room if 3 tablets do not relieve the pain.
   d. Take nitroglycerin only if resting for 5 minutes does not relieve the pain.

4. Mr. Lynch began using a long-acting nitroglycerin patch, Nitro-Dur, 2 days ago. He complains of a severe headache during this time. The nurse should:
   a. Suggest applying the patch at bedtime.
   b. Tell Mr. Lynch that acetaminophen should relieve the headache.
   c. Advise him to wait 1 hour after removing the old patch before applying a new one.
   d. Report the headache to the physician immediately.

5. Propranolol (Inderal) is prescribed for 55-year-old Martin Evers to prevent angina. Mr. Evers should be taught to:
   a. Place the tablet between his cheek and gum.
   b. Take a dose prior to performing any activity that is likely to induce angina.
   c. Schedule doses 1 hour before or 2 hours after meals.
   d. Lie down for 1 hour after taking each dose.

6. The client who is taking nifedipine (Procardia) should be told to report which of the following to the physician?
   a. Urinary frequency
   b. Swelling of feet or ankles
   c. Muscle rigidity
   d. Mental depression

7. Mrs. Adams is taking procainamide (Procan SR), 500 mg QID. The drug will have to be discontinued if she develops drug-induced systemic lupus. Signs of systemic lupus include:
   a. Pain in finger joints, fever, and dyspnea.
   b. Tinnitus, vertigo, and light-headedness.
   c. Pallor and numbness of hands, muscle pain, and visual changes.
   d. Hyperventilation, tinnitus, diaphoresis, and vomiting.

8. Mrs. Abel, who has congestive heart failure, is admitted to the hospital for treatment of digitalis toxicity. Her electrocardiogram shows frequent premature ventricular contractions. The nurse should expect to administer which antiarrhythmic drug?
   a. Quinidine
   b. Phenytoin
   c. Propranolol
   d. Verapamil

9. Mrs. Perry's hypertension has been successfully controlled with clonidine (Catapres) for 3 years. When she becomes depressed after her husband's death, amitriptyline (Elavil) is started to relieve her depression. She will need to be monitored for:
   a. Respiratory depression.
   b. Dehydration.
   c. An increase in blood pressure.
   d. Peripheral neuropathy.

10. An appropriate nursing diagnosis for the client taking hydralazine (Apresoline) to treat hypertension would be:

   a. Fluid volume deficit related to diuretic effects of drug.
   b. Sleep pattern disturbance related to CNS stimulation.
   c. Constipation related to slowed peristalsis.
   d. Potential for injury related to orthostatic hypotension.

11. Which of the following laboratory test alterations is common in clients receiving captopril (Capoten)?

   a. Protein in the urine
   b. Glucose in the urine
   c. Decreased serum potassium
   d. Increased serum sodium

12. Evelyn Albert has an acute attack of glaucoma. Mannitol (Osmitrol) is ordered to help decrease her intraocular pressure. Before administering the mannitol, the nurse must check:

   a. Apical pulse.
   b. Urine output.
   c. Serum potassium.
   d. Serum glucose.

ANSWERS

1. Correct answer is a. Visual changes, such as shimmering, yellowing, or halos around objects are signs of digitalis toxicity.

   b. Hearing assessment would detect ototoxicity, which is not a common sign of digitalis toxicity. Ototoxicity occurs with loop diuretics.
   c. Urine output assessment would detect nephrotoxicity, which is not a common sign of digitalis toxicity.
   d. Gait changes would be seen with peripheral neuropathy or cerebellar effects. Neither is common with digitalis toxicity.

2. Correct answer is d. Hypokalemia increases the risk of digitalis toxicity. It is important to consume adequate dietary potassium to minimize the risk.

   a. Treatment of congestive heart failure usually includes sodium restriction. Increasing dietary sodium would promote fluid retention, antagonizing the therapeutic effects of digitalis.
   b. Pyridoxine is increased to reduce the risk of peripheral neuropathy. Digitalis does not cause this problem.
   c. Calcium levels are not altered by digitalis, so there is no reason to increase dietary calcium.

3. Correct answer is c. If 3 tablets taken 5 minutes apart do not relieve the pain, it is probably not anginal pain. Since it could be a myocardial infarction, prompt medical attention is indicated.

   a. Nitroglycerin tablets need to be protected from heat and light, but refrigeration is not needed.
   b. Since nitroglycerin's duration of action is very short, there is no daily dose limit.
   d. Nitroglycerin should be taken as soon as pain is experienced. The client should also rest to reduce cardiac demand, but delaying drug administration serves no purpose.

4. Correct answer is b. Headache is a common side effect of transdermal nitroglycerin that usually diminishes as tolerance develops. A mild analgesic may be used to relieve the pain until tolerance develops.

   a. Changing the time for applying the patch would have no effect on occurrence of side effects, since transdermal absorption maintains a steady plasma level of the drug.
   c. Waiting 1 hour would not affect occurrence of side effects. Some clients develop tolerance to the therapeutic effects rapidly. Keeping the patch off prevents this. Usually the patch is removed at bedtime and reapplied in the morning.
   d. Headache is a common side effect, not a toxic effect. It would only be necessary to consult the physician if ordinary measures to relieve the headache did not work.

5. **Correct answer is c.** Propranolol should be taken on an empty stomach for maximum effectiveness. Food delays absorption.

   a. Propranolol is taken PO, not by the buccal route.

   b. Taking a dose prior to an activity likely to cause angina is an appropriate use of nitroglycerin. Propranolol is taken on a regular schedule to achieve its preventive effect.

   d. Lying down is indicated when severe postural hypotension is anticipated at the time of peak effect, as with the first dose of nitrates. This is not true of propranolol.

6. **Correct answer is b.** Peripheral edema may be a sign of fluid volume excess secondary to congestive heart failure. The myocardial depressant action of calcium channel blockers can precipitate or exacerbate congestive heart failure.

   a. Urinary frequency is not a side effect of calcium channel blockers.

   c. Calcium channel blockers may cause cramping of muscles, but muscle rigidity is not an anticipated side effect.

   d. Mental depression is not an effect of calcium channel blockers, although it does occur with some beta-blockers.

7. **Correct answer is a.** Drug-induced systemic lupus mimics many of the symptoms of the disease lupus erythematosus. Although the characteristic butterfly rash is often absent, pain in small joints, pleuritic pain, dyspnea, fever, and blood dyscrasias do occur.

   b. Tinnitus, vertigo, and light-headedness are symptoms of quinidine toxicity.

   c. Pallor, hand numbness, muscle pain, and visual changes are symptoms of toxicity of the ergot alkaloids used to treat migraine headache.

   d. Hyperventilation, tinnitus, diaphoresis, and vomiting are symptoms of salicylism, or aspirin toxicity.

8. **Correct answer is b.** Phenytoin is the drug of choice to manage digitalis-induced arrhythmias.

   a. Quinidine can increase the risk of digitalis toxicity when the 2 drugs are given together. It is not used to manage digitalis-induced arrhythmias.

   c and **d.** Because beta-adrenergic blockers and calcium channel blockers can induce or exacerbate congestive heart failure, they are usually avoided in clients with that disorder unless the benefits outweigh the risks.

9. **Correct answer is c.** Tricyclic antidepressants antagonize the blood-pressure-reducing effects of central adrenergic inhibitors. Since the therapeutic effect of clonidine is blocked, the blood pressure can be expected to rise.

   a. Neither clonidine nor amitriptyline causes respiratory depression.

   b. Dehydration is unlikely. Both drugs cause dry mouth, which can cause the client to consume excessive amounts of fluid. Clonidine can cause fluid retention.

   d. Neither drug is neurotoxic, so peripheral neuropathy is not a major concern.

10. **Correct answer is d.** All antihypertensive drugs can cause orthostatic hypotension.

    a. Vascular smooth muscle relaxants often cause fluid retention and are usually given with diuretics for that reason.

    b. Sedation is the expected effect of antihypertensive drugs.

    c. Vascular smooth muscle relaxants act specifically on vascular smooth muscle. They do not alter peristalsis. Diarrhea is a more likely side effect.

11. **Correct answer is a.** Proteinuria, especially during the first few months of therapy, is common.

    b. Captopril does not alter blood glucose levels. Since glucose in urine appears when serum glucose is high, it would not be expected with captopril.

    c. Hyperkalemia is a side effect of captopril. Hypokalemia would be seen with diuretics.

    d. Serum sodium levels are not affected by captopril.

12. **Correct answer is b.** Before administering an osmotic diuretic, the nurse must be certain renal function is adequate to excrete the drug. A history of oliguria or anuria may signal renal impairment. If mannitol is not excreted, its effect is prolonged, and increased blood pressure or congestive heart failure may occur.

a. Apical rate is checked before administration of digitalis, calcium channel blockers, or beta-adrenergic blockers. It is not an essential baseline assessment for mannitol.

c. Mannitol is not a potassium-wasting diuretic, so it is less likely to cause hypokalemia than thiazide or loop diuretics.

d. Although mannitol is a sugar, it is not metabolized in the body, so it will not alter serum glucose.

6

Drugs Affecting the Respiratory System

OVERVIEW

I. Antitussive, expectorant, and mucolytic agents
- A. Antitussive agents
- B. Expectorant agents
- C. Mucolytic agents
- D. Nursing diagnoses
- E. Nursing implementation factors
- F. Nursing evaluations

II. Bronchodilators
- A. Sympathomimetics
- B. Xanthine derivatives
- C. Nursing diagnoses
- D. Nursing implementation factors
- E. Nursing evaluations

III. Antiasthmatic prophylactics
- A. Cromolyn sodium
- B. Corticosteroids
- C. Nursing diagnoses
- D. Nursing implementation factors
- E. Nursing evaluations

IV. Antihistamines
- A. Examples
- B. Use/mechanism of action
- C. Adverse effects
- D. Contraindications
- E. Precautions
- F. Drug interactions
- G. Nursing diagnoses
- H. Nursing implementation factors
- I. Nursing evaluations

V. Oxygen therapy
- A. Examples
- B. Use/mechanism of action
- C. Adverse effects
- D. Contraindications
- E. Precautions
- F. Drug interactions
- G. Nursing diagnoses
- H. Nursing implementation factors
- I. Nursing evaluations

NURSING HIGHLIGHTS

1. The nurse should always remember that even minor difficulty in breathing provokes great anxiety and requires reassurance and explanation.
2. The nurse should emphasize lifestyle changes such as stopping smoking and practicing relaxation techniques that may have a long-term effect on reducing respiratory distress in clients with disorders such as asthma and emphysema.

iodism—chronic poisoning by iodine or iodides; symptoms include angioedema, laryngeal edema, cutaneous and mucosal hemorrhage, and serum sickness

mucolytic—an agent that causes mucus to disintegrate

ENHANCED OUTLINE

I. Antitussive, expectorant, and mucolytic agents

See text pages
_____

A. Antitussive agents
  1. Examples: benzonatate (Tessalon), codeine, dextromethorphan hydrobromide (Robitussin-DM), hydrocodone bitartrate (Hycodan), diphenhydramine (Benadryl)
  2. Use/mechanism of action: suppress coughing by altering response threshold of cough center in the medulla or peripherally by inhibiting pulmonary stretch, thus decreasing impulses to the cough center
  3. Adverse effects
     a) Benzonatate: dizziness, sedation, headache, gastrointestinal (GI) upset, constipation, skin rash
     b) Dextromethorphan: adverse effects including drowsiness and GI upset; toxic reactions including euphoria, hyperactivity, nystagmus, uncoordinated movements, stupor, shallow breathing
     c) Codeine (at antitussive doses): adverse effects including impaired alertness or coordination, hypersensitivity, dependence (with long-term use); toxic reactions including miosis, bradycardia, tachycardia, hypotension, narcosis, seizures, circulatory collapse, respiratory arrest
     d) Hydrocodone bitartrate: dizziness, sedation, nausea, vomiting
  4. Contraindications: pregnancy, lactation, known hypersensitivity
  5. Precautions: benign prostatic hypertrophy, debilitation, thoracotomy, laparotomy, history of drug abuse
  6. Drug interactions
     a) Benzonatate: no significant drug interactions
     b) Dextromethorphan and MAO (monoamine oxidase) inhibitors: excitation, hyperpyrexia
     c) Narcotic antitussives with MAO inhibitors, alcohol, and other central nervous system (CNS) depressants: potentiation of CNS depressive effects
     d) Hydrocodone bitartrate and MAO inhibitors: excitation, hypertension or hypotension, coma

B. Expectorant agents
  1. Examples: guaifenesin (Robitussin), iodinated glycerol (Organidin), potassium iodide (Pima), terpin hydrate
  2. Use/mechanism of action: facilitate expulsion of mucus by reducing adhesiveness and surface tension of mucus

       3. Adverse effects (see Nurse Alert, "Signs and Symptoms of Iodism")
         a) Guaifenesin: vomiting at high doses
         b) Iodides: thyroid disease with prolonged use; iodism; aggravation of acne
         c) Terpin hydrate: drowsiness
       4. Contraindications: pregnancy, lactation, known hypersensitivity; thyroid disease (with iodinated glycerin)
       5. Precautions: respiratory insufficiency, inadequate cough reflex
       6. Drug interactions
         a) Guaifenesin and oral anticoagulants: increased risk of bleeding
         b) Iodides and lithium or antithyroid agents: potentiation of hypothyroid effects, goiter
         c) Terpin hydrate and disulfiram: alcohol-disulfiram reaction

   C. Mucolytic agents
       1. Examples: acetylcysteine (Mucomyst)
       2. Use/mechanism of action: enhance mucolysis by altering molecular composition of mucus, reducing viscosity
       3. Adverse effects: nausea, stomatitis, hypersensitivity, and bronchospasm
       4. Contraindications: known hypersensitivity
       5. Precautions: pregnancy, lactation, asthma, advanced age or debilitation combined with respiratory insufficiency
       6. Drug interactions
         a) Amphotericin, erythromycin, ampicillin: inactivation of these agents
         b) Acetaminophen (overdose): alteration of metabolic pathway of acetaminophen when used with activated charcoal

   D. Nursing diagnoses
       1. Ineffective airway clearance related to respiratory disorder
       2. Fluid volume deficit related to diarrhea
       3. Potential for infection related to buildup of respiratory secretions
       4. Potential for injury related to CNS depression

   E. Nursing implementation factors
       1. Administration procedures
         a) Increase fluid intake of client taking expectorant.

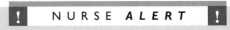

! NURSE ALERT !

Signs and Symptoms of Iodism

Long-term or high-dose use of iodide-containing expectorants can cause iodism. Signs and symptoms of iodism are unpleasant brassy taste, burning in mouth and throat, sore gums, increased salivation, coryza, sneezing, and eye irritation. Early symptoms may be mistaken for a common cold.

      b) Do not administer terpin hydrate to an alcoholic or a person suspected of being an alcoholic.

  2. Daily monitoring and measurements

      a) Monitor client taking codeine for signs of respiratory depression.

      b) Monitor iodide expectorant client for signs of iodism, hyperthyroidism, and iodide toxicity.

  3. Points for client teaching

      a) Caution client about terpin hydrate's high alcohol content.

      b) Explain to client the importance of increasing fluid intake when taking an expectorant.

      c) Encourage patient who is confined to bed and taking an expectorant to turn, breathe deeply, and cough every 2 hours.

      d) Warn client taking a narcotic antitussive not to drink alcohol.

      e) Caution client that prolonged use of codeine may cause dependence.

      f) Show client how to use and clean nebulizer for acetylcysteine administration.

      g) Teach client using iodide expectorant the signs and symptoms of iodism and iodine sensitivity and advise client to report any symptoms to physician.

F. Nursing evaluations

  1. Client shows absence of coughing.

  2. Client shows improved ability to cough up mucus.

  3. Client has no signs or symptoms of infection.

  4. Client shows no signs of excessive CNS depression.

II. Bronchodilators (sympathomimetics, xanthine derivatives) (see Client Teaching Checklist, "How to Use an Inhaler")

See text pages
_____

A. Sympathomimetics

  1. Examples: epinephrine (Bronkaid Mist, Asthmahaler, Asthma Nefrin); isoproterenol (Vapo-Iso, Isuprel); isoetharine (Bronkosol, Bisorine); albuterol (Proventil, Ventolin); terbutaline (Brethaire, Brethine)

  2. Use/mechanism of action: treat asthma, bronchitis, and emphysema by acting on bronchial smooth muscle to produce bronchodilation

  3. Adverse effects: same as section V,C of Chapter 3

  4. Contraindications: same as section V,D of Chapter 3

  5. Precautions: same as section V,E of Chapter 3

  6. Drug interactions: same as section V,F of Chapter 3

B. Xanthine derivatives

  1. Examples: theophylline (Bronkodyl, Elixophyllin); aminophylline; dyphylline (Dilor); oxtriphylline (Choledyl)

  2. Use/mechanism of action: treat asthma, bronchitis, and emphysema by inhibiting mast cell degranulation and histamine release

  3. Adverse effects: nausea, anxiety, restlessness; toxic reactions including insomnia, headaches, behavior changes, irritability, severe nausea, cramps, convulsions, tachycardia, irregular heartbeat, rapid breathing

  4. Contraindications: known hypersensitivity

       5. Precautions: advanced age, congestive heart failure, liver impairment, peptic ulcers, acute myocardial injury, cardiac arrhythmias, severe hypoxemia, hypertension, hyperthyroidism, diabetes, benign prostatic enlargement

       6. Drug interactions

         a) Phenytoin, primidone, rifampin: increased xanthine metabolism; decreased phenytoin absorption

         b) Beta-blockers: cause mutual inhibition; decreased theophylline excretion

         c) Cimetidine, ranitidine, erythromycin, troleandomycin: decreased theophylline metabolism, possible toxicity

         d) Tobacco, marijuana: increased theophylline metabolism

C. Nursing diagnoses

    1. Ineffective airway clearance related to pulmonary disorder

    2. Activity intolerance related to pulmonary disorder

    3. Potential for injury related to irritation of mucous membranes

    4. Anxiety related to diagnosis

D. Nursing implementation factors

    1. Administration procedures

       a) Administer xanthine derivatives slowly, intravenously (IV).

       b) Do not mix xanthine drugs with epinephrine, norepinephrine, isoproterenol, or penicillin G.

       c) Administer oral xanthine drugs on an empty stomach unless GI irritation occurs.

       d) Measure blood levels when administering aminophylline by continuous infusion.

✔ CLIENT TEACHING CHECKLIST ✔

How to Use an Inhaler

Teach the client with asthma the following approach to using an inhaler. Demonstrate first with a placebo inhaler and then have client repeat the process until learned.

1. Insert canister into plastic shell, remove cap, and shake unit.
2. Exhale fully, until it feels as though no more air can be exhaled.
3. Place mouthpiece in mouth with lips firmly closed.
4. Place top of canister between forefinger and thumb while inhaling deeply.
5. Hold inhaled breath as long as possible.
6. Release pressure on canister, remove unit from mouth, and breathe slowly.

2. Daily monitoring and measurements
    a) Observe client for signs of theophylline toxicity, including hypotension, tachycardia, ventricular arrhythmias, and convulsions.
    b) Use pulmonary studies or respiratory parameters such as FEV_1 and TV to monitor therapeutic effect.
3. Points for client teaching
    a) Caution theophylline client not to take over-the-counter (OTC) drugs containing ephedrine or other sympathomimetics and provide him/her with examples of such drugs.
    b) Tell theophylline client to limit consumption of caffeine beverages and charcoal-broiled foods, since charcoal increases theophylline elimination.
    c) Explore factors that cause breathing attacks and teach holistic measures to reduce stress and encourage coping.
    d) Advise elderly clients that they may experience dizziness while taking xanthine derivatives.
    e) Warn client of danger of tolerance, drug toxicity, and paradoxical airway resistance with overuse of sympathomimetic bronchodilator.

E. Nursing evaluations
    1. Client achieves therapeutic effects and avoids adverse effects.
    2. Client reports easier breathing.
    3. Client reports greater activity tolerance.
    4. Client avoids respiratory infection.
    5. Client's anxiety is relieved.

III. Antiasthmatic prophylactics

See text pages
_____

A. Cromolyn sodium
    1. Example: cromolyn sodium (Intal)
    2. Use/mechanism of action: prevent bronchospasms and bronchial asthma attacks by inhibiting release of histamine and leukotrienes from mast cells
    3. Adverse effects: sneezing, watering of eyes, dizziness, nausea, rash, headache, increased urgency and frequency of urination
    4. Contraindications: lactose intolerance, cardiac arrhythmias, coronary artery disease
    5. Precautions: renal or hepatic impairment, lactation
    6. Drug interactions: none reported

B. Corticosteroids
    1. Examples: beclomethasone (Vanceril, Beclovent); dexamethasone (Decadron); ipratropium (Atrovent)
    2. Use/mechanism of action: prevent bronchospasms and bronchial asthma attacks by suppressing antibodies that precipitate asthmatic attack
    3. Adverse effects
        a) Short-term effects: dry mouth, hoarseness, cough, headache, nausea, bronchial spasm; oral candidiasis or monilial esophagitis (with beclomethasone)
        b) Effects from prolonged systemic use: osteoporosis, adrenal hypercorticism, cataracts, stunted growth in children

4. Contraindications: status asthmaticus, nonasthmatic bronchial disorders
5. Precautions: tuberculosis, ocular herpes simplex, untreated systemic infections
6. Drug interactions: limited with aerosol administration; more extensive with systemic steroids

C. Nursing diagnoses
   1. Ineffective airway clearance related to pulmonary disorder
   2. Altered urinary elimination patterns related to adverse effects of cromolyn therapy
   3. Altered comfort related to disagreeable taste of inhalant

D. Nursing implementation factors
   1. Administration procedures
      a) Check integrity of client's nasal and oral airways before and after bronchodilator therapy.
      b) Administer a bronchodilator, if one is to be used, 15 minutes before beclomethasone inhalation.
   2. Daily monitoring and measurements
      a) Monitor respiratory patterns and pulse rate and rhythm in client taking bronchodilator.
      b) Examine mouth of client taking beclomethasone for signs of infection.
   3. Points for client teaching
      a) Suggest that client rinse mouth after bronchodilator inhalation to alleviate bad taste of medication.
      b) Show client how to use a nebulizer.
      c) Tell client that a month of consistent compliance may be necessary before full benefits of bronchodilators are achieved.

E. Nursing evaluations
   1. Client achieves good therapeutic response without adverse effects.
   2. Client resumes normal urinary elimination pattern.
   3. Client minimizes unpleasant taste of medication by rinsing mouth and gargling.

See text pages

IV. Antihistamines

A. Examples: brompheniramine (Dimetane), chlorpheniramine (Chlor-Trimeton), dimenhydrinate (Dramamine), terfenadine (Seldane), astemizole (Hismanal), diphenhydramine (Benadryl)

B. Use/mechanism of action: treat allergies, vertigo, and motion sickness by competing with histamine for H_1 receptors in smooth muscle of vascular system and bronchiole, lacrimal, salivary, and respiratory mucosal glands

C. Adverse effects: drowsiness, dry mouth, blurred vision, blood dyscrasias, hypotension, confusion

D. Contraindications: MAO inhibitor therapy

E. Precautions: asthma, benign prostatic hypertrophy, narrow-angle glaucoma, advanced age

F. Drug interactions: potentiation of CNS depressive and/or anticholinergic effects when taken with alcohol, CNS depressants, anticholinergics, MAO inhibitors

G. Nursing diagnoses
    1. Ineffective airway clearance related to respiratory disorder
    2. Urinary retention related to anticholinergic effects of medication
    3. Fluid volume deficit related to anticholinergic effects of medication
    4. Potential for injury related to drowsiness
    5. Potential for infection related to buildup of bronchial secretions

H. Nursing implementation factors
    1. Administration procedures
        a) For motion sickness, antihistamines should be taken 30 minutes to 2 hours before they are needed.
        b) To minimize gastric upset, antihistamines should be taken with food or milk.
    2. Daily monitoring and measurements
        a) Take periodic blood counts when antihistamines are used for long-term therapy.
        b) Monitor client for signs and symptoms of blood dyscrasia, including sore throat, fever, unusual bruising or bleeding, and exhaustion.
    3. Points for client teaching
        a) Tell client not to break, crush, or chew sustained-release capsules or long-acting tablets.
        b) Tell client to practice good dental hygiene if he/she is using antihistamines on a long-term basis, since they can contribute to caries and gum disease.

I. Nursing evaluations
    1. Client's airways are clear.
    2. Client resumes normal urinary patterns.
    3. Client achieves normal hydration.
    4. Client restricts potentially dangerous activities while taking medication.
    5. Client has no signs or symptoms of infection.

V. Oxygen therapy

A. Examples: oxygen administered through nasal catheter or cannula, mask, or tent

See text pages

B. Use/mechanism of action: treat dyspnea by reversing hypoxia and hypoxemia

C. Adverse effects (rare): oxygen toxicity, including substernal pain, increased respiratory distress, nausea, vomiting, restlessness, tremors, twitching, paresthesias, convulsions, dry hacking cough

D. Contraindications: none

E. Precautions
1. Risk of oxygen-induced hypoventilation in chronic obstructive pulmonary disease
2. Risk of retrolental fibroplasia in premature infants

F. Drug interactions: increased potential for oxygen toxicity in clients receiving high concentrations of oxygen on long-term basis if also receiving adrenocorticotropic hormone (ACTH), aspirin, atropine, carbon dioxide inhalation, dextroamphetamine, insulin, thyroid preparations

G. Nursing diagnoses
1. Impaired gas exchange related to altered oxygen supply
2. Anxiety related to difficulty in breathing
3. Potential for injury related to oxygen toxicity

H. Nursing implementation factors
1. Administration procedures
   a) If a nasal catheter is used to administer oxygen, clean or replace it several times a day.
   b) To avoid drying mucous membranes, ensure that nasally administered oxygen is humidified if 4 l/minute or more are being used.
2. Daily monitoring and measurements
   a) Monitor vital signs.
   b) Observe level of consciousness and skin color and temperature for any abnormalities.
   c) Evaluate arterial blood gas levels and measure pulse oximetry.
3. Points for client teaching
   a) Caution client and family about the danger of smoking when oxygen is being administered.
   b) Explain the hazards of open flames, electric appliances, oils, wool blankets, alcohol, and other flammable liquids near client or oxygen tank.

I. Nursing evaluations
1. Client demonstrates improved ventilation.
2. Client remains calm, with anxiety reduced to manageable level.
3. Client's blood gases are within normal limits.

1. To increase the effectiveness of the expectorant guaifenesin (Robitussin), the client should be taught to:

   a. Gargle frequently with an antimicrobial mouthwash.
   b. Maintain a semi-Fowler's position.
   c. Drink at least 8 glasses of water daily.
   d. Maintain bed or chair rest until the cough subsides.

2. An appropriate nursing diagnosis to address side effects of the mucolytic drug acetylcysteine (Mucomyst) would be:

   a. Altered oral mucous membranes related to irritation by the drug.
   b. Fluid volume deficit related to altered electrolyte balance.
   c. Diarrhea related to smooth muscle stimulant effects.
   d. Altered thought processes related to sulfur toxicity.

3. James Boggs, who has chronic obstructive pulmonary disease (COPD), will be using a nebulizer to self-administer acetylcysteine (Mucomyst) at home. He should be taught to:

   a. Discard any solution that has turned lavender.
   b. Refrigerate opened medication containers.
   c. Sterilize the nebulizer equipment by boiling for 20 minutes after each use.
   d. Schedule the last treatment of the day at least 2 hours before bedtime.

4. Albuterol (Ventolin) 2 puffs every 4 hours by inhaler is prescribed for Margaret Good, who suffers from chronic bronchitis. The most effective way to administer this dose is to:

   a. Administer both puffs during 1 prolonged inhalation.
   b. Administer 1 puff, take a deep breath, then administer a second puff.
   c. Administer 1 puff, wait 5 minutes, then administer a second puff.
   d. Administer 1 puff while lying on the left side, then administer a second puff while lying on the right side.

5. A side effect commonly reported by elderly clients taking terbutaline (Brethine) orally is:

   a. Cold hands and feet.
   b. Urinary retention.
   c. Fluid volume excess.
   d. Oversedation.

6. Mr. Fulmer, who smoked 2 packs of cigarettes a day for 30 years, has been stabilized on theophylline (Theo-Dur) to manage his chronic bronchitis. Mr. Fulmer now reports that he has stopped smoking. The nurse should anticipate:

   a. Shorter duration of therapeutic effects of theophylline.
   b. Decreased therapeutic effect of theophylline.
   c. Symptoms of theophylline toxicity.
   d. Fewer adverse effects of theophylline.

7. Mr. Barnes's serum theophylline level is reported as 27 mcg/ml (therapeutic range 10–20 mcg/ml) and his theophylline is discontinued. What is the most important action for the nurse to take until the theophylline level drops?

   a. Have equipment available for respiratory support.
   b. Initiate seizure precautions.
   c. Take appropriate safety precautions for excessive sedation.
   d. Prepare to administer a diuretic for fluid overload.

8. After using her cromolyn sodium (Intal) inhaler for a week, Mrs. Alton reports that she has seen no improvement in her asthmatic symptoms. The nurse should:

   a. Explain that it takes several weeks to achieve therapeutic effects.
   b. Assess Mrs. Alton for use of caffeinated beverages.
   c. Consult the physician about a dosage increase.
   d. Suggest that she see the physician for reevaluation, as she may need a different drug.

9. Before cromolyn sodium (Intal) by turbo inhaler is prescribed, the client should be assessed for:

   a. Seafood allergy.
   b. History of arrhythmias.
   c. History of glaucoma.
   d. Lactose intolerance.

10. An appropriate nursing diagnosis to address adverse effects of an antihistamine is:

    a. Urge incontinence related to increased reactivity of bladder muscle.
    b. Fluid volume excess related to sodium retention.
    c. Ineffective airway clearance related to thickened secretions.
    d. Sleep pattern disturbance related to central nervous system (CNS) stimulation.

11. It is appropriate to administer hydrocodone bitartrate (Hycodan) syrup:

    a. Every 2 hours.
    b. Before meals.
    c. Before percussion and postural drainage.
    d. Before nebulizer or aerosol therapy.

12. Diphenhydramine (Benadryl) 25 mg IM stat is ordered to treat an acute drug-induced dystonia. The nurse should:

    a. Use Z-track technique to administer the drug.
    b. Apply ice to the site for 5 minutes before injecting the drug.
    c. Use the deltoid site for drug injection.

    d. Question an order to inject an antihistaminic drug.

ANSWERS

1. **Correct answer is c.** Increased oral fluid intake provides the extra fluid necessary to produce thinner secretions that are more easily cleared by ciliary movement and the cough reflex.

   a. Antimicrobial mouthwashes are often alcohol based. Alcohol dries the mucous membranes of the throat, which may cause an irritating dry cough.
   b. Maintaining any one position would permit secretions to pool. The client should change position frequently to help mobilize secretions.
   d. Immobility promotes pooling of secretions. Mild exercise encourages deep breathing, which helps mobilize and clear secretions.

2. **Correct answer is a.** If mouth care is not given soon after the nebulizer treatment, the acetylcysteine may damage oral mucosa, causing stomatitis.

   b. Acetylcysteine does not cause electrolyte balance alterations or affect fluid balance.
   c. Acetylcysteine has no effect on smooth muscle motility.
   d. Acetylcysteine may cause drowsiness but does not alter thought processes. If altered thought processes occur, the client should be assessed for problems with oxygenation.

3. **Correct answer is b.** Acetylcysteine solution does not contain a preservative and must therefore be refrigerated once the container is opened.

   a. It is not necessary to discard solution that turns lavender. This is a common alteration that does not affect drug potency.
   c. Sterilization of the equipment is not necessary. It can be cleaned by washing with a mild dish detergent and hot water and air-drying in a clean place.
   d. Drowsiness is a common side effect of acetylcysteine and scheduling a treatment

at bedtime minimizes the impact of this effect. In addition, if secretions are liquefied and cleared at bedtime, the client may obtain a longer period of undisturbed sleep.

4. **Correct answer is c.** The 5-minute wait allows the first puff to dilate the upper airways so the second puff can reach the lower airways.

   a and b. Administering both puffs during 1 prolonged inhalation or administering 1 puff, taking a deep breath, and administering another puff would not provide adequate time for the first puff to dilate upper airways so that the second puff could act on lower airways.
   d. Lying on the side does not permit full lung expansion, impairing an even delivery of medication throughout the airways.

5. **Correct answer is a.** The peripheral vasoconstriction that results from adrenergic drug effects frequently leads to coldness or tingling in the extremities, especially in the elderly.

   b. Urinary urgency or urge incontinence, not urinary retention, is the most likely effect.
   c. Hypervolemia is unlikely. Adrenergic effects generally strengthen cardiac contraction and produce mild diuresis.
   d. The elderly are very sensitive to the CNS stimulant effects of adrenergics and often manifest confusion or anxiety. Sedation would be unusual.

6. **Correct answer is c.** Mr. Fulmer's dosage was based on the 4- to 5-hour half-life of theophylline in smokers. Because he has stopped smoking, the half-life will return to the normal 7–8 hours. Since theophylline has a narrow therapeutic range, toxicity is very likely to develop.

   a. Smoking shortens the duration of effect. Because Mr. Fulmer has quit smoking, therapeutic effects can be expected to last longer.
   b. As the half-life lengthens, the therapeutic effect can be expected to increase.
   d. As the half-life lengthens, adverse effects can be expected to increase.

7. **Correct answer is b.** Seizures are a known toxic effect of theophylline. While Mr. Barnes's theophylline level is elevated, he is at high risk for a seizure.

   a. Respiratory arrest is not a common toxic effect of theophylline.
   c. Sedation is unlikely. Toxic effects of theophylline involve CNS stimulation and include anxiety, irritability, and insomnia.
   d. Fluid overload is unlikely. Theophylline has mild diuretic effects, and toxicity may cause vomiting or diarrhea, all of which would lead to fluid volume deficit.

8. **Correct answer is a.** Cromolyn sodium is only minimally absorbed into cell membranes, so it often takes several weeks for therapeutic effects to appear.

   b. There are no known drug interactions with cromolyn sodium, since its action is topical rather than systemic.
   c and d. Seeking a dosage increase or a reevaluation of the client would be premature. Full therapeutic effect cannot be assessed until several weeks of daily dosing have passed. Increasing the dosage or changing drugs should not be considered until the full effect of the cromolyn sodium can be evaluated.

9. **Correct answer is d.** The powder in the capsules used in the turbo inhaler has a lactose base. Clients with lactose intolerance should receive the metered dose inhaler form of cromolyn sodium. Since lactose intolerance is very common among African-American and Asian individuals, it is especially important to question them about this problem.

   a. Assessment for seafood allergy would be appropriate for medications containing iodine but does not apply to cromolyn.
   b. Assessment for a history of arrhythmias would be important for the metered-dose form of the drug, since the propellant can exacerbate arrhythmias.
   c. Glaucoma is a contraindication for some bronchodilators but does not apply to cromolyn.

10. **Correct answer is c.** Antihistamines dry nasal mucosa and increase viscosity of respiratory secretions. While this effect relieves the watery nasal discharge of colds or hay fever, it may cause individuals with chronic obstructive pulmonary disease (COPD) or other respiratory disorders to have increased difficulty mobilizing the more tenacious secretions.

   a. Urge incontinence is seen with drugs that have cholinergic effects. Antihistamines are strongly anticholinergic.
   b. Fluid volume deficit, not excess, is the common side effect of antihistamines, due to adverse GI effects such as nausea, vomiting, and diarrhea.
   d. Sedation is a common side effect of antihistamines. This nursing diagnosis would be more appropriate for bronchodilators.

11. **Correct answer is b.** Hydrocodone bitartrate is a cough suppressant. Since clients with respiratory problems often avoid eating or drinking because it stimulates coughing, administration of a cough suppressant before meals may improve the client's nutritional status.

a. Hydrocodone bitartrate should be administered only every 4–6 hours. Giving it every 2 hours would lead to overdose.
c and d. Percussion and postural drainage and nebulizer or aerosol therapy are intended to mobilize respiratory secretions. An effective cough is necessary to clear these secretions. A cough suppressant should not be administered until the client has had a chance to remove the mobilized secretions by coughing.

12. **Correct answer is a.** Antihistamines are irritating to subcutaneous tissue. Z-track technique should be used to prevent the medication from leaking back into subcutaneous tissue.

   b. While applying ice would decrease the pain of antihistamine injection, it would also delay absorption. In an emergency situation, when the drug is ordered stat, any action that delays absorption is contraindicated.
   c. The deltoid is a relatively small muscle mass and should not be used for very irritating drugs such as antihistamines.
   d. Although the usual route for antihistamines is oral, they may be given IM in emergency situations.

7

Drugs Affecting the Gastrointestinal System

NURSING HIGHLIGHTS

1. The nurse should teach client the fundamentals of good diet as the long-term solution to many gastrointestinal problems.
2. Many clients assume that over-the-counter antacids, laxatives, and similar remedies cannot do harm and consequently use them without restraint. In taking the client history, the nurse should question client to identify excessive or inappropriate use of these agents.
3. The nurse should question client with a peptic ulcer about nonsteroidal anti-inflammatory drug (NSAID) use.

I. Antacids	II. Histamine$_2$-receptor antagonists and other peptic ulcer agents	III. Antidiarrheal agents and laxatives	IV. Emetic and antiemetic agents

See text pages
_____

GLOSSARY

chemoreceptor trigger zone—the part of the medulla that stimulates the vomiting center to begin emesis after receiving sensory information from the stomach and other parts of the body

hyperaluminemia—accumulation of aluminum in lungs, bones, and nerve tissue caused by use of aluminum-containing antacids in clients with renal failure; may lead to dementia and osteomalacia

hypermagnesemia—accumulation of magnesium in the body caused by the use of magnesium-containing antacids in clients with renal failure; symptoms include nausea and vomiting, electrocardiogram changes, hypotension, respiratory or mental depression, and coma

hyperphosphatemia—accumulation of phosphates in the body caused by long-term use of aluminum-containing antacids; symptoms include malaise, muscle weakness, and anorexia

hypoperistalsis—decreased waves of contractions in the large intestine; symptoms include anorexia, nausea, abdominal distention, and absence of bowel sounds and bowel movements

milk-alkali syndrome—a condition caused by the chronic administration of sodium bicarbonate with milk and other calcium-containing products, characterized by hypercalcemia, crystalluria, renal insufficiency, and tissue calcification

ENHANCED OUTLINE

I. Antacids

A. Examples: aluminum/magnesium compounds (Aludrox, Maalox, Mylanta); sodium bicarbonate (Alka-Seltzer); calcium carbonate (Tums); magnesium hydroxide (Milk of Magnesia)

B. Use/mechanism of action: treat hyperacidity associated with peptic ulcer, gastritis, peptic esophagitis, gastric hyperacidity, heartburn, and hiatal hernia by buffering or neutralizing stomach acid

C. Adverse effects (see Client Teaching Checklist, "Antacids," and Nurse Alert, "Milk-Alkali Syndrome")
  1. Aluminum antacids: constipation, phosphate depletion, renal stones, encephalopathy, bone demineralization
  2. Sodium bicarbonate: systemic alkalosis, acid rebound
  3. Calcium antacids: milk-alkali syndrome, renal stones, acid rebound, constipation, decreased phosphate levels
  4. Magnesium antacids: diarrhea, hypokalemia, hypermagnesemia

D. Contraindications: renal dysfunction, known hypersensitivity

E. Precautions: gastric outlet syndrome, renal impairment

F. Drug interactions
  1. Ketoconazole with antacids: decreased ketoconazole absorption
  2. Mecamylamine with antacids: decreased mecamylamine excretion
  3. Methenamine with antacids: decreased effectiveness of methenamine
  4. Oral tetracyclines with antacids: formation of chemical complex that decreases tetracycline absorption
  5. Digitalis drugs with antacids: decreased digitalis absorption
  6. Ion-exchange resin with calcium or magnesium antacids: systemic alkalosis
  7. Phenothiazine with magnesium antacids or aluminum hydroxide: decreased phenothiazine absorption
  8. Isoniazid with aluminum antacids: decreased isoniazid absorption

G. Nursing diagnoses
  1. Pain related to gastric disorder
  2. Potential for injury related to gastric disorder

H. Nursing implementation factors
   1. Administration procedures
      a) Avoid giving other oral medications within 1–2 hours of antacid administration, because antacid may interfere with absorption.
      b) Refrain from administering antacids within 1 hour of enteric medication, since antacids may cause premature drug release.
   2. Daily monitoring and measurements
      a) Monitor long-term aluminum antacid client for signs of hyperaluminemia, including osteomalacia and dementia, and for signs of hypophosphatemia, including anorexia, muscle weakness, and malaise.
      b) Monitor client for changes in bowel patterns.
   3. Points for client teaching
      a) Advise client with renal failure to prevent hypermagnesemia by avoiding the use of magnesium antacids.
      b) Caution client on sodium-restricted diets to avoid antacids with a high sodium content.
      c) Tell client who must restrict potassium intake to check antacid labels and avoid products with a high potassium content.
      d) Teach patient the recommended schedule for taking antacids.

I. Nursing evaluations
   1. Client's pain is relieved.
   2. Client makes dietary changes to achieve long-term management of hyperacidity.

II. Histamine$_2$-receptor antagonists and other peptic ulcer agents

See text pages
_____

A. H$_2$ agonists
   1. Examples: cimetidine (Tagamet), ranitidine (Zantac), famotidine (Pepcid), nizatidine (Axid)
   2. Use/mechanism of action: treat peptic ulcer disease, Zollinger-Ellison syndrome, and GI reflux disease; prevent stress ulcers by binding competitively to H$_2$ receptors, reducing acid secretion
   3. Adverse effects: headache, nausea, skin rash, impotence, neutropenia, gynecomastia, constipation, diarrhea; confusion, agitation, hallucinations in elderly or debilitated clients; severe bradycardia with rapid IV administration
   4. Contraindications: lactation, known hypersensitivity
   5. Precautions: pregnancy, renal or hepatic impairment
   6. Drug interactions
      a) Antacids: inhibition of absorption of H$_2$ antagonists
      b) Oral anticoagulants, propranolol, benzodiazepines, tricyclic antidepressants, theophylline, procainamide, quinidine, lidocaine,

phenytoin, calcium channel blockers, cyclosporine, carbamazepine, narcotic analgesics: inhibition of hepatic metabolism by cimetidine, increasing drug serum levels and risking toxicity
- c) Carmustine: increased bone marrow toxicity caused by cimetidine
- d) Alcohol: decreased metabolism and increased absorption by cimetidine

B. Other peptic ulcer agents
1. Examples: sucralfate (Carafate), misoprostol (Cytotec), omeprazole (Prilosec)
2. Use/mechanism of action: treat peptic ulcer disease and prevent stress ulcers and NSAID-induced ulcers by acting as a prostaglandin (misoprostol) or a proton pump inhibitor (omeprazole) or by forming a barrier at ulcer site, helping it to heal (sucralfate)
3. Adverse effects: gastrointestinal (GI) upset (misoprostol); headache, GI upset, dizziness, rash (omeprazole); constipation (sucralfate)
4. Contraindications: known hypersensitivity
5. Precautions: renal dysfunction, pregnancy, lactation
6. Drug interactions
   - a) Diazepam, phenytoin, and warfarin: increased half-lives of these drugs with omeprazole, heightening risk of toxicity
   - b) Ketoconazole, ampicillin esters, iron salts: altered pH, reducing absorption, caused by omeprazole
   - c) Sucralfate: decreased bioavailability of cimetidine

C. Nursing diagnoses
1. Impaired tissue integrity related to peptic ulcer
2. Pain related to peptic ulcer

D. Nursing implementation factors
1. Administration procedures
   - a) Avoid giving antacid within 1 hour of H_2 antagonist administration.
   - b) Dilute cimetidine in at least 50 ml, famotidine in at least 100 ml, and ranitidine in at least 20 ml of compatible IV solution before IV administration, using saline, 5% or 10% dextrose, lactated Ringers, or 5% sodium bicarbonate.
2. Daily monitoring and measurements
   - a) Monitor client for signs of cardiovascular toxicity, such as severe bradycardia, while administering H_2 antagonist by infusion.
   - b) Check complete blood count (CBC) for abnormalities in client receiving cimetidine.
3. Points for client teaching
   - a) Advise client not to take antacid within 1 hour of an H_2 antagonist dose.
   - b) Suggest that client prevent constipation by increasing fiber and fluid intake.
   - c) Warn client that H_2 antagonist might impair alertness and balance, and that he/she should avoid operating dangerous machinery until effects are known.

E. Nursing evaluations
1. Client reports decrease or absence of pain and nausea.
2. Client experiences reduction of gastric acid secretion.

III. Antidiarrheal agents and laxatives

See text pages

A. Antidiarrheal agents
1. Examples: opium tincture, paregoric, difenoxin (Motofen), diphenoxylate (Lomotil), loperamide (Imodium), kaolin/pectin mixtures (Kaopectate)
2. Use/mechanism of action: treat diarrhea by decreasing stomach motility and peristalsis (opium tincture and paregoric); decreasing peristalsis (difenoxin, diphenoxylate, loperamide); or binding with bacteria and other irritants on intestinal mucosa (kaolin and pectins)
3. Adverse effects: (see Nurse Alert, "Hypoperistalsis")
    a) Opium tincture and paregoric: nausea, vomiting, constipation
    b) Difenoxin, diphenoxylate, loperamide: nausea, vomiting, abdominal discomfort, central nervous system (CNS) depression, tachycardia, hypoperistalsis, paralytic ileus
    c) Kaolin and pectins: occasional constipation
4. Contraindications
    a) Opium tincture and paregoric: known hypersensitivity
    b) Difenoxin, diphenoxylate, loperamide: known hypersensitivity, antibiotic-induced diarrhea, pseudomembranous colitis
    c) Kaolin and pectins: none reported
5. Precautions
    a) Opium tincture and paregoric: asthma, drug abuse, liver or kidney dysfunction, pregnancy, lactation
    b) Difenoxin, diphenoxylate, loperamide: benign prostate hypertrophy, liver or kidney impairment, pregnancy, lactation
    c) Kaolin and pectins: none
6. Drug interactions
    a) Opium tincture and paregoric, difenoxin, diphenoxylate, loperamide: enhanced depressant effects of alcohol, barbiturates, tranquilizers, and other CNS depressants

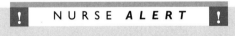

! NURSE *ALERT* !

Hypoperistalsis

Monitor clients using difenoxin, diphenoxylate, or loperamide to treat diarrhea for signs and symptoms of hypoperistalsis. These include anorexia, nausea, abdominal distention, and absence of bowel sounds, flatus, and bowel movements.

b) Kaolin and pectins: interference with absorption of lincomycin or digoxin if administered concurrently

B. Laxatives
1. Examples: glycerin; lactulose (Cephulac, Chronulac); magnesium salts (Milk of Magnesia); sodium biphosphate/phosphate (Fleet Enema, PhosphoSoda); docusate (Surfak, Kasof, Dialose, Regutol); bisacodyl (Dulcolax); castor oil; phenolphthalein (Ex-Lax); senna (X-Prep); bulk-forming laxatives (Cologel, Citrucel, Maltsupex, FiberCon, Mitrolan, Metamucil, Syllact, Konsyl-D, Correctol); mineral oil
2. Use/mechanism of action: treat constipation by
   a) Causing fluid retention and distention in the intestine, promoting evacuation (glycerin, lactulose, magnesium salts, sodium biphosphate/phosphate)
   b) Softening stools by emulsifying fecal fat and water (docusate)
   c) Encouraging peristalsis by irritating intestinal mucosa or stimulating smooth muscle of intestine (bisacodyl, castor oil, phenolphthalein, senna)
   d) Increasing fecal bulk and water content, stimulating peristalsis and evacuation (fiber and bulk-forming laxatives)
   e) Acting as a lubricant, preventing colon from absorbing water from stool (mineral oil)
3. Adverse effects
   a) Glycerin, lactulose, magnesium salts, sodium biphosphate/phosphate: fluid and electrolyte imbalances
   b) Docusate: occasional cramping
   c) Bisacodyl, castor oil, phenolphthalein, senna: weakness, nausea, abdominal cramps
   d) Fiber and bulk-forming laxatives: flatulence
   e) Mineral oil: nausea, vomiting, diarrhea, abdominal cramping
4. Contraindications
   a) Glycerin, lactulose, magnesium salts, sodium biphosphate/phosphate, fiber and bulk-forming laxatives: none reported
   b) Docusate: renal dysfunction
   c) Bisacodyl, castor oil, phenolphthalein, senna: intestinal obstruction, lactation, acute abdominal disease
   d) Mineral oil: advanced age, debilitation, pregnancy, hiatal hernia
5. Precautions
   a) Glycerin, lactulose, magnesium salts, sodium biphosphate/phosphate, fiber and bulk-forming laxatives, mineral oil: none
   b) Docusate: pregnancy, lactation
   c) Bisacodyl, castor oil, phenolphthalein, senna: pregnancy
6. Drug interactions
   a) Glycerin, lactulose, magnesium salts, sodium biphosphate/phosphate, fiber, and bulk-forming laxatives: no significant interactions
   b) Docusate: increased absorption of oral drugs; systemic absorption of mineral oil
   c) Bisacodyl, castor oil, phenolphthalein, senna: possible reduced absorption of oral drugs administered concurrently

d) Mineral oil: hindering of absorption of fat-soluble vitamins, oral contraceptives, anticoagulants; reduction of antibacterial activity of sulfonamides

C. Nursing diagnoses
   1. Fluid volume deficit related to diarrhea
   2. Diarrhea-related infectious disorder
   3. Pain related to abdominal cramping

D. Nursing implementation factors
   1. Administration procedures
      a) Administer bulk-forming laxatives with at least 8 oz of fluid to avoid esophageal obstruction.
      b) Avoid administering mineral oil with orally absorbed drugs.
   2. Daily monitoring and measurements
      a) Monitor hydration in clients with diarrhea.
      b) Monitor client receiving opium antidiarrheal and another CNS depressant for increased CNS depression.
      c) Monitor client receiving difenoxin or diphenoxylate, which contain atropine, for signs of atropine toxicity.
      d) Monitor client using difenoxin, diphenoxylate, or loperamide for signs and symptoms of hypoperistalsis.
   3. Points for client teaching
      a) Advise client not to self-medicate for diarrhea for more than 48 hours, but to contact physician if problem persists.
      b) Caution client to avoid alcohol and other CNS depressants during therapy with difenoxin, diphenoxylate, or loperamide.
      c) Teach client the signs of atropine toxicity, hypoperistalsis, and toxic megacolon, as appropriate.
      d) Warn client to avoid laxative dependence.
      e) Tell client to discontinue laxative and contact physician if rash or pruritus occurs.
      f) Teach client how to maintain regular bowel elimination pattern.

E. Nursing evaluations
   1. Client maintains normal hydration.
   2. Client achieves therapeutic effect and has normal elimination.
   3. Client's pain is eliminated.

IV. Emetic and antiemetic agents

See text pages

A. Emetic agents
   1. Examples: ipecac syrup, apomorphine
   2. Use/mechanism of action: treat ingestion of toxic substances by the induction of vomiting through stimulation of vomiting center of medulla or chemoreceptor trigger zone (CTZ)

3. Adverse effects: euphoria, restlessness, tachypnea, tremors, CNS depression, orthostatic hypotension
4. Contraindications: seizures, shock, eating disorders, ingestion of petroleum products
5. Precautions: lactation, pregnancy, arteriosclerosis, atherosclerosis
6. Drug interactions: rare, since used in acute cases

B. Antiemetic agents
1. Examples
    a) Antihistamines: buclizine (Bucladin-S), cyclizine (Marezine), dimenhydrinate (Dramamine), diphenhydramine (Benadryl), hydroxyzine hydrochloride (Ataraz), meclizine (Antivert), trimethobenzamide (Tigan)
    b) Phenothiazines: chlorpromazine (Thorazine), perphenazine (Trilafon), prochlorperazine (Compazine), promethazine (Phenergan), thiethylperazine (Torecan)
    c) Benzquinamide (Emete-con), scopolamine (Transderm Scōp), metoclopramide (Reglan), diphenidol (Vontrol), dronabinol (Marinol)
2. Use/mechanism of action: control nausea and vomiting caused by vertigo, motion sickness, and drug adverse effects by inhibiting vestibular system; exerting anticholinergic or CNS depressant effects; suppressing vomiting center; blocking dopamine receptors (phenothiazine)
3. Adverse effects (see Nurse Alert, "Hypoperistalsis")
    a) Antihistamine antiemetics: drowsiness, paradoxic CNS stimulation in children, mild anticholinergic effects
    b) Phenothiazine antiemetics: sedation, hypotension, extrapyramidal reactions (rare at antiemetic doses), anticholinergic effects
    c) Benzquinamide: sedative, anticholinergic effects
    d) Scopolamine: anticholinergic effects
    e) Diphenidol: anticholinergic effects, hallucinations, confusion, disorientation
4. Contraindications
    a) Antihistamine antiemetics: lactation, known hypersensitivity, neonatal status
    b) Phenothiazine antiemetics: CNS depression, bone marrow depression, brain damage, known hypersensitivity
    c) Benzquinamide, scopolamine, diphenidol: same as other anticholinergics (see section IV,D of Chapter 3)
5. Precautions
    a) Antihistamine antiemetics: seizures, glaucoma, benign prostatic hypertrophy, asthma, cardiac arrhythmias, pregnancy
    b) Phenothiazine antiemetics: hepatic, respiratory, or cardiovascular disease; hypocalcemia, seizures, glaucoma, benign prostatic hypertrophy
    c) Benzquinamide, scopolamine, diphenidol: same as other anticholinergics (see section IV,E of Chapter 3)

6. Drug interactions
   a) Antihistamine antiemetics
      (1) CNS depressants: additive CNS depression
      (2) Anticholinergics: additive anticholinergic effects
      (3) Ototoxic drugs: masked ototoxicity
   b) Phenothiazine antiemetics
      (1) Guanethidine: inhibition of guanethidine uptake
      (2) Amphetamine, anxiolytics: mutual inhibition
      (3) Anticholinergics: increased anticholinergic effects and decreased antiemetic effects
      (4) Barbiturates: increased CNS depression
      (5) Levodopa: decreased antiparkinsonian effects
      (6) Lithium: increased risk of neurotoxicity and encephalopathy; respiratory depression and hypotension
      (7) Droperidol: increased risk of extrapyramidal effects

C. Nursing diagnoses
   1. Potential for injury related to vomiting
   2. Fluid volume deficit related to vomiting
   3. Altered oral mucous membranes related to dehydration
   4. Altered nutrition, less than body requirements, related to vomiting

D. Nursing implementation factors
   1. Administration procedures
      a) Consult poison control center to confirm that induction of vomiting is appropriate therapy for substance ingested.
      b) Refrain from administering second dose of apomorphine if vomiting does not occur with first dose.
      c) Administer second dose of ipecac syrup if vomiting does not occur within 30 minutes.
      d) Administer antihistamines with food or milk to avoid gastric upset.
   2. Daily monitoring and measurements
      a) Monitor client receiving antiemetic for adverse anticholinergic effects.
      b) Monitor pediatric client receiving antihistamines for paradoxic CNS stimulation, including restlessness, insomnia, euphoria, tremor, and seizures.
   3. Points for client teaching
      a) Explain the purpose of the poison control center and provide client with local telephone number.
      b) Teach client how and when to use ipecac syrup to induce vomiting in cases of poisoning.
      c) Tell motion sickness client to take drug 30–60 minutes before beginning activity expected to cause sickness.

       d) Caution client using scopolamine patches to avoid touching the drug side of the patch and to wash hands after application, as transferring drug from hand to eye can cause pupil dilatation.

E. Nursing evaluations
   1. Client reports absence of vomiting and decrease of nausea.
   2. Client maintains normal hydration.
   3. Client's mucous membranes remain intact.
   4. Client has induced emesis.

1. An appropriate nursing diagnosis to address common side effects of aluminum-based antacids used to decrease the pain of gastritis is:

   a. Constipation related to gastrointestinal (GI) effects of aluminum.

   b. Diarrhea related to GI effects of aluminum.

   c. Altered thought processes related to central nervous system (CNS) effects of aluminum.

   d. Fluid volume deficit related to adverse GI effects of antacid.

2. The nurse should recognize that the infusion rate of IV cimetidine is too rapid if the client experiences:

   a. Tremors.

   b. Dyspnea.

   c. Sedation.

   d. Bradycardia.

3. Mr. Thomas takes theophylline to control his asthma. When he develops a duodenal ulcer, his physician prescribes cimetidine 300 mg QID. The nurse should monitor Mr. Thomas for which drug interaction?

   a. Cimetidine toxicity

   b. Reduced effectiveness of cimetidine

   c. Theophylline toxicity

   d. Reduced effectiveness of theophylline

4. Sucralfate (Carafate) is prescribed to treat Mrs. Proctor's peptic ulcer. Mrs. Proctor asks what the drug is supposed to do for her. The best response by the nurse is:

   a. "It will neutralize the acid in your stomach."

   b. "It will reduce your stomach's acid production."

   c. "It will form a protective coating over the ulcer."

   d. "It will reduce peristalsis to prevent irritation of the ulcer."

5. Mrs. Davis, 27 years old, takes large doses of a nonsteroidal anti-inflammatory drug (NSAID) for rheumatoid arthritis. Misoprostol (Cytotec) is prescribed to prevent NSAID-induced ulcers. The nurse should tell her:

   a. To use an alternative contraceptive method if she has been taking oral contraceptives.

   b. To avoid becoming pregnant while taking misoprostol.

   c. That her menses may be lighter than usual while she is taking misoprostol.

   d. That misoprostol blocks ovulation and will have to be stopped if she wants to conceive.

6. Diphenoxylate (Lomotil) and loperamide (Imodium) are contraindicated for clients with:

   a. Antibiotic-induced diarrhea.

   b. Congestive heart failure.

   c. Diarrhea caused by hyperosmotic tube-feeding solutions.

   d. Fecal incontinence.

7. Ann Maxwell is given kaolin/pectin (Kaopectate) to treat diarrhea secondary to gastroenteritis. She should be warned that:

   a. She may have increased abdominal cramps after taking kaolin/pectin.

   b. She should watch for distention or failure to pass flatus.

   c. She should not drive or operate machinery for 3–4 hours after taking kaolin/pectin.

   d. Her stools will be white or pale for 1–2 days after taking kaolin/pectin.

8. When administering a bulk-forming laxative such as Metamucil to an elderly client, it is especially important for the nurse to:

   a. Avoid administering other medications within 2 hours.

   b. Be sure that the client drinks 8 oz of fluid with the medication.

   c. Determine that the client has adequate renal function before administering the medication.

d. Assess electrolyte balance frequently after giving the medication.

9. The best nursing diagnosis to address the side effects of a hyperosmolar laxative such as magnesium hydroxide would be:

   a. Altered nutrition, less than body requirements, related to malabsorption of fat-soluble vitamins.
   b. Anxiety related to red discoloration of urine.
   c. Fluid volume deficit related to intestinal losses via osmotic effects.
   d. Altered oral mucous membranes related to irritation by the medication.

10. To promote the desired emetic effect of syrup of ipecac, the nurse should administer it with:

    a. 8 oz water.
    b. 4 oz orange juice.
    c. 8 oz milk.
    d. Activated charcoal solution.

11. Administration of an emetic would be indicated for which of the following clients?

    a. A teenager who acts drunk after rapid consumption of a large amount of beer
    b. A woman who attempted suicide by swallowing a bottle of sleeping pills and does not respond to verbal stimuli
    c. A 4-year-old child who ate an unknown quantity of baby aspirin
    d. An elderly man who has been self-treating arthritis with large doses of ibuprofen and shows signs of toxicity

12. Six-year-old Tonya is admitted with a 2-day history of vomiting due to gastroenteritis. The antihistamine antiemetic trimethobenzamide (Tigan) is ordered for her. After administering the drug, the nurse should monitor Tonya for signs of:

    a. Fluid overload.
    b. Nephrotoxicity.
    c. Hepatotoxicity.
    d. Excessive central nervous system stimulation.

---

1. **Correct answer is a.** Aluminum is very constipating. With long-term use, the client should be encouraged to increase fluid and fiber intake.

   b. A diagnosis of diarrhea related to GI effects would be appropriate for a magnesium-based antacid. Magnesium has laxative effects.
   c. Altered thought processes would reflect aluminum toxicity, which occurs only with prolonged use of large doses, such as with a renal failure client who might take the antacid to control high phosphate levels.
   d. Aluminum-based antacids do not induce vomiting or diarrhea, which might lead to fluid volume deficits.

2. **Correct answer is d.** Too-rapid IV infusion of cimetidine can cause severe bradycardia and other symptoms of cardiac toxicity.

   a and **b.** Tremors and dyspnea are not symptoms of cimetidine toxicity. They may be seen during infusion of xanthines or other bronchodilators.
   c. Confusion and agitation may occur in elderly clients receiving IV cimetidine, but sedation is unlikely.

3. **Correct answer is c.** Cimetidine inhibits hepatic metabolism of many drugs, increasing the serum drug levels and thus heightening the risk of toxicity. This is a particular risk with theophylline, which has a narrow therapeutic range.

   a and **b.** Theophylline does not alter the metabolism of cimetidine.
   d. Inhibited metabolism of drugs would increase the serum drug level. Higher drug levels would not decrease the therapeutic effect.

4. **Correct answer is c.** Sucralfate reacts with the protein in the ulcer's exudate to form a coating over the ulcer. This prevents

---

acid and digestive enzymes from worsening the ulceration.

a. Neutralizing stomach acid describes the action of an antacid.

b. Reduction of stomach acid production describes the action of a histamine$_2$-receptor antagonist.

d. Reduction of peristalsis describes the action of an anticholinergic.

5. **Correct answer is b.** Misoprostol can induce miscarriages if taken during pregnancy.

a. Misoprostol does not alter the effectiveness of oral contraceptives. It is important that Mrs. Davis use an effective form of contraception while taking misoprostol.

c. Since prostaglandins can increase uterine contractions, cramping or hypermenorrhea are more likely than decreased menstrual flow.

d. Misoprostol does not affect ovulation. An effective form of contraception should be used while taking it.

6. **Correct answer is a.** Antibiotic-induced diarrhea may be caused by the overgrowth of bacteria in the intestine. Drugs that slow peristalsis increase the risk that these organisms may penetrate the intestinal mucosa and cause more serious infections.

b. Antidiarrheals do not have adverse cardiac effects, so this is not a contraindication.

c. Osmotic diarrhea is one of the problems for which antidiarrheals may be used.

d. There is no reason to avoid antidiarrheals when the client is incontinent. Incontinent clients are at greater risk for skin breakdown due to diarrhea.

7. **Correct answer is d.** Kaolin is a fine white clay that makes the stools light or white in color.

a. Increased abdominal cramps would occur if peristalsis were speeded up. Since kaolin/pectin does not speed peristalsis, this is not an anticipated effect.

b. Distention cautions are appropriate for drugs that slow peristalsis, such as loperamide, diphenoxylate, or paregoric. These are symptoms of hypoperistalsis, which is not a concern with kaolin/pectin.

c. Sedation is common with loperamide, diphenoxylate, and paregoric, so this warning would be appropriate for them. It is unnecessary for kaolin/pectin, since it is not absorbed systemically.

8. **Correct answer is b.** If the client does not drink adequate fluid to flush all medication out of the esophagus, it may swell and create esophageal obstruction. This is especially important with the elderly, who have a less efficient swallowing function than younger adults.

a. Withholding other medications for 2 hours is unnecessary, as bulk-forming laxatives have no significant interactions. It would be appropriate for bisacodyl, castor oil, or senna.

c. Bulk-forming laxatives are not systemically absorbed and therefore are not excreted via the kidneys. This would be appropriate for docusate.

d. Frequent assessment of electrolyte balance would be appropriate for magnesium salts (Milk of Magnesia) or sodium biphosphate (Fleet enema), which can cause electrolyte imbalances. Metamucil does not affect electrolytes.

9. **Correct answer is c.** Hypovolemia is a serious and common side effect of hyperosmolar laxatives. They draw large amounts of fluid into the intestinal lumen. If this fluid is not replaced by oral intake, a deficit develops. With repeated laxative use, the deficit may progress to hypovolemic shock.

a. A diagnosis of altered nutrition, less than body requirements, would be appropriate for a lubricant laxative such as mineral oil. Fat-soluble vitamins dissolve in the mineral oil, which is then excreted, carrying the vitamins with it. Hyperosmolar laxatives do not have this effect.

b. Anxiety related to urine discoloration would be appropriate for a stimulant laxative such as phenolphthalein, cascara, or senna, which may cause red or red-brown discoloration of urine. Hyperosmolar laxatives do not have this effect.

d. The hyperosmolar laxatives do not irritate mucous membranes, so altered oral mucosa would be unlikely.

10. **Correct answer is a.** For maximum effect, syrup of ipecac must be administered with sufficient water to distribute it throughout the stomach, promoting contact with as large an area of gastric mucosa as possible in the shortest possible time. Diluting the stomach contents liquefies them, making them easier to expel.

    b. Four oz would be an inadequate amount of fluid. An acidic juice would cause esophageal burning when it is vomited, increasing client discomfort.

    c. There would be no specific reason to use milk as the liquid with which to administer syrup of ipecac. Clear liquids provide the maximum effect.

    d. Activated charcoal would adsorb the syrup of ipecac, preventing its desired effect.

11. **Correct answer is c.** Emetics are commonly used to remove ingested toxic substances from the stomach before they can be absorbed. When the history of the overdose is known and it is known or suspected that a large volume of drug was recently ingested, an emetic is appropriate.

    a. Emetics are contraindicated in severe inebriation.

    b. Emetics are contraindicated when the client may become unconscious soon. When the possibility of loss of gag reflex exists, the risk of aspiration is too great to permit emetic use.

    d. The history suggests that this is a case of chronic poisoning, in which case the drug has already been systemically absorbed and an emetic will be of no use.

12. **Correct answer is d.** Although sedation is a common side effect of antihistamines in adults, paradoxic stimulation is not uncommon in children. Restlessness, tremors, and insomnia are early signs.

    a. Fluid retention is not a common side effect of antihistamines. Although dry mouth may occur and may increase thirst, the fluid intake would be needed to counteract losses related to vomiting and would not cause an excess.

    b and c. Neither nephrotoxicity nor hepatotoxicity is a common effect of antihistamines.

8

Drugs Affecting the Endocrine and Reproductive Systems

OVERVIEW

I. Thyroid and antithyroid agents
  A. Thyroid agents
  B. Antithyroid agents
  C. Nursing diagnoses
  D. Nursing implementation factors
  E. Nursing evaluations

II. Parathyroid agents
  A. Examples
  B. Use/mechanism of action
  C. Adverse effects
  D. Contraindications
  E. Precautions
  F. Drug interactions
  G. Nursing diagnoses
  H. Nursing implementation factors
  I. Nursing evaluations

III. Corticosteroids
  A. Glucocorticoids
  B. Mineralocorticoids
  C. Nursing diagnoses
  D. Nursing implementation factors
  E. Nursing evaluations

IV. Antidiabetic therapy
  A. Insulin
  B. Oral hypoglycemic agents
  C. Nursing diagnoses

  D. Nursing implementation factors
  E. Nursing evaluations

V. Pituitary hormones
  A. Anterior pituitary agents
  B. Posterior pituitary agents
  C. Nursing diagnoses
  D. Nursing implementation factors
  E. Nursing evaluations

VI. Male and female hormonal agents
  A. Androgens
  B. Anabolic steroids
  C. Estrogens and progestins
  D. Nursing diagnoses
  E. Nursing implementation factors
  F. Nursing evaluations

VII. Drugs affecting labor and lactation
  A. Uterine-stimulating agents
  B. Uterine-inhibiting (tocolytic) agents
  C. Lactation suppressants
  D. Nursing diagnoses
  E. Nursing implementation factors
  F. Nursing evaluations

1. Since hormonal therapy can cause disturbing alterations in appearance and sexual functioning, the nurse should advise the client that doses can be adjusted to reduce these effects, which are usually reversible, and that he/she should report adverse effects rather than stopping therapy.
2. The nurse should advise the client when a newly prescribed drug may affect libido or sexual performance; the nurse should give client the time and privacy to raise such issues and show openness to listening to sexual concerns and problems.
3. The nurse should encourage a client newly diagnosed with diabetes by explaining that he/she can look forward to a full life with little impairment if all instructions about good hygiene and foot care, diet, exercise, and prescribed medication are followed carefully.

GLOSSARY

antidiuretic hormone (ADH)—a water-conserving hormone that concentrates and decreases urine output; synthesized in the hypothalamus and stored in the posterior pituitary gland, it is also called vasopressin

diabetic ketoacidosis—acidosis due to the accumulation of ketone bodies that occurs in clients with insulin-dependent diabetes mellitus; symptoms include fatigue, deep and rapid fruity breathing, confusion, hypotension, greatly increased urine output followed by oliguria or anuria, and coma

hyperthyroidism—excessive thyroid gland activity, also called thyrotoxicosis, characterized by increased metabolic rate and disturbances in the autonomic nervous system and in creatine metabolism; symptoms and signs include prominent eyes; thin, fine hair; intolerance to heat; and hot, moist skin

hypothyroidism—deficient thyroid gland activity, characterized by decreased metabolic rate; symptoms and signs include edematous eyelids; dry, brittle hair; intolerance to cold; and cold, dry skin

thyroid-stimulating hormone (TSH)—a hormone, also called thyrotropin, that is released by the anterior pituitary gland and controls the growth and functioning of the thyroid gland

thyrotropin-releasing hormone (TRH)—a hormone released by the hypothalamus that controls the levels of thyrotropin in the body

ENHANCED OUTLINE

I. Thyroid and antithyroid agents

A. Thyroid agents
  1. Examples: thyroid USP (desiccated); levothyroxine (Levothroid, Noroxine, Synthroid); liothyronine (Cytomel); liotrix (Euthroid); thyroglobulin (Proloid); thyrotropin (TSH); protirelin (Relefact-TRH)
  2. Use/mechanism of action: treat hypothyroidism by functioning as natural or synthetic hormones containing triiodothyronine and/or thyroxine

See text pages

3. Adverse effects: diarrhea, abdominal cramps, weight loss, increased appetite, palpitations, tachycardia, hypertension, angina, arrhythmias, headache, tremor, insomnia, fever, heat intolerance, menstrual cycle irregularities
4. Contraindications: thyrotoxicosis, acute myocardial infarction, uncorrected adrenal insufficiency, known hypersensitivity
5. Precautions: angina, hypertension, advanced age, lactation
6. Drug interactions
   a) Oral anticoagulants: increased risk of bleeding
   b) Cholestyramine, colestipol: binding to thyroid hormones
   c) Phenytoin, carbamazepine: increased metabolism of thyroid hormones
   d) Cardiac glycosides: decreased digitoxin or digoxin serum levels
   e) Theophylline: decreased theophylline serum levels

B. Antithyroid agents
   1. Examples
      a) Thioamides: methimazole (thiamazole), propylthiouracil (PTU)
      b) Iodides: iodine, radioactive iodine (^{131}I), SSKI

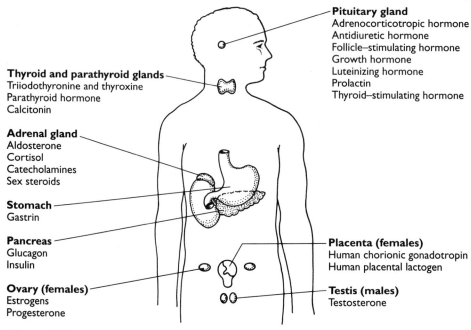

Figure 8–1
Glands and Hormones of the Endocrine System

2. Use/mechanism of action: treat hyperthyroidism by interfering with hormone synthesis, modifying tissue response to thyroid hormones, or destroying the thyroid gland
3. Adverse effects: nausea, vomiting, decreased appetite, hepatitis, headache, drowsiness, dizziness, irregular menses, nephritis, joint and muscle pain, hyperpigmentation, hair loss, lymphadenopathy; granulocytopenia (thioamides); iodism (iodides)
4. Contraindications: lactation, known hypersensitivity
5. Precautions: tuberculosis, concurrent therapy with another drug causing granulocytopenia (e.g., clozapine)
6. Drug interactions: synergistic hypothyroidism with iodide and lithium

C. Nursing diagnoses
1. Altered nutrition, less (or more) than body requirements, related to thyroid dysfunction
2. Sleep pattern disturbance related to thyroid dysfunction
3. Altered activity level related to thyroid dysfunction

D. Nursing implementation factors
1. Administration procedures
   a) Avoid abrupt withdrawal of a thyroid drug from client with myxedema, because doing so may cause myxedema coma.
   b) Notify physician immediately if client taking thyroid agent develops chest pain.
   c) Advise client taking ^{131}I to take precautions at home, especially around children, because urine, saliva, perspiration, and vomit will be radioactive for 7 days.
2. Daily monitoring and measurements
   a) Closely monitor client taking thyroid agent for signs of toxicity.
   b) Check complete blood count (CBC) regularly during antithyroid therapy.
   c) Observe client taking an iodide for signs of iodism.
   d) Monitor client taking antithyroid agent for signs of hypothyroidism, including depression, cold intolerance, and edema.
3. Points for client teaching
   a) Teach client receiving thyroid therapy the signs of toxicity (headaches, palpitations, and nervousness) and of hyperthyroidism (fatigue, dyspnea, and heat intolerance).
   b) Warn client taking thioamide to call physician immediately if sore throat and fever occur.
   c) Advise client to wait several months after radioactive iodine therapy before becoming pregnant or fathering a child.

E. Nursing evaluations
1. Client achieves therapeutic effects and avoids adverse effects of thyroid agent.
2. Client consumes food within normal limits to compensate for weight loss or gain caused by thyroid agent.
3. Client resumes normal sleep pattern.
4. Client resumes normal level of activity.

See text pages

II. Parathyroid agents

A. Examples: calcitonin-salmon (Calcimar), etidronate (Didronel), calcifediol (Calderol), calcitriol (Rocaltrol), dihydrotachysterol (DHT)

B. Use/mechanism of action: treat calcium disorders such as Paget's disease, hypercalcemia of infancy, hypocalcemia of various etiologies, vitamin D intoxication, and postmenopausal osteoporosis by exerting hypocalcemic effects, thus reducing bone resorption (calcitonin and etidronate), or by raising serum calcium through promotion of calcium absorption (calcifediol, calcitriol, dihydrotachysterol)

C. Adverse effects
   1. Calcitonin: flushing, nausea, vomiting, urticaria
   2. Etidronate: GI distress (infrequent)
   3. Vitamin D analogues: vitamin D intoxication, whose signs, in order of appearance, include weakness, fatigue, headache, nausea, vomiting, diarrhea; polyuria, polydipsia, nocturia; kidney stones; osteoporosis

D. Contraindications: lactation, hypercalcemia, vitamin D toxicity

E. Precautions: pregnancy, renal impairment, digitalis therapy

F. Drug interactions
   1. Calcitonin with theophylline, isoproterenol: increased bone resorption
   2. Etidronate with drugs containing calcium, iron, magnesium, or aluminum: decreased etidronate absorption
   3. Calcifediol with cholestyramine, colestipol: decreased calcifediol absorption
   4. Calcifediol with thiazide diuretics: hypercalcemia in hypoparathyroidism clients

G. Nursing diagnoses
   1. Pain related to suppressed bone mineralization
   2. Altered health maintenance related to vitamin D intoxication

H. Nursing implementation factors
   1. Administration procedures
      a) Perform skin allergy test before administering calcitonin.
      b) Take seizure precautions, such as padded bed rails, with hypocalcemic client.
   2. Daily monitoring and measurements
      a) Monitor serum calcium level.
      b) Check for signs of hypocalcemic tetany.
   3. Points for client teaching
      a) Teach client to recognize signs and symptoms of hypocalcemia during calcium regulator therapy and of hypercalcemia if he/she is

receiving vitamin D analogue (see Client Teaching Checklist, "Hypocalcemia and Hypercalcemia").
    b) Instruct client to report any sudden, unexplained bone pain.
I. Nursing evaluations
    1. Client's pain is decreased.
    2. Client's calcium levels are within normal limits.
    3. Client's vitamin D level is within normal limits.

III. Corticosteroids

A. Glucocorticoids
    1. Examples: beclomethasone (Beclovent, Vanceril); betamethasone (Celestone); cortisone (Cortone); dexamethasone (Decadron); hydrocortisone (Cortef, Hydrocortone)
    2. Use/mechanism of action: treat adrenocortical insufficiency and inflammatory and immune reactions by suppression of hypersensitivity and immune response
    3. Adverse effects (see Client Teaching Checklist, "Corticosteroid Therapy")
        a) Central nervous system (CNS): mood swings, insomnia, seizures
        b) Endocrine/metabolic: increased blood sugar, hyperlipidemia, adrenal atrophy, Cushingoid symptoms; dysmenorrhea; altered protein, fat, and carbohydrate metabolism; protein catabolism (see Nurse Alert, "Cushingoid Signs and Symptoms")

See text pages

✔ CLIENT TEACHING CHECKLIST ✔

Hypocalcemia and Hypercalcemia

Teach a client receiving parathyroid therapy the following signs of hypocalcemia and hypercalcemia:

Signs of hypocalcemia:

✔ Cardiac arrhythmias and arrest
✔ Chvostek's sign (twitching of the legs or cheeks evoked by tapping or stroking the area over the facial nerve in front of the ear)
✔ Facial spasms and grimace
✔ Laryngospasm
✔ Neuromuscular irritability
✔ Seizures
✔ Tetany

Signs of hypercalcemia:

✔ Cardiac arrhythmias
✔ Drowsiness
✔ Exhaustion and muscle weakness
✔ Headache
✔ Constipation
✔ Metallic taste in mouth

---

      c) Immune system: increased susceptibility to infection, suppression of signs and symptoms of infection

      d) Musculoskeletal: osteoporosis, aseptic bone necrosis, muscle wasting, myopathy, arthralgia

      e) GI: peptic ulcer, pancreatitis

      f) Cardiovascular: hypertension, edema, thrombophlebitis, embolism, atherosclerosis

      g) Other: hirsutism, glaucoma, cataracts, buffalo hump

4. Contraindications: systemic fungal infection, known hypersensitivity

5. Precautions: peptic ulcers, renal disease, hypertension, osteoporosis, diabetes, hypothyroidism, seizures, congestive heart failure, serious infection

6. Drug interactions

      a) Barbiturates, phenytoin, rifampin, aminoglutethimide: increased corticosteroid metabolism, reducing effectiveness

      b) Amphotericin B, chlorthalidone, ethacrynic acid, furosemide, thiazide-type diuretics: increased risk of hypokalemia

      c) Erythromycin, troleandomycin: decreased corticosteroid metabolism

      d) Salicylates: increased risk of peptic ulcers; decreased plasma levels of salicylates

      e) NSAIDs: increased risk of peptic ulcers

✔ CLIENT TEACHING CHECKLIST ✔

Corticosteroid Therapy

Discuss the following precautions and information with a client receiving corticosteroid therapy:

✔ Avoid using limb for 24–48 hours if drug has been injected intra-articularly.

✔ Report any signs of infection, including fever, sore throat, and delayed wound healing.

✔ Avoid immunization while taking corticosteroids.

✔ Report any visual disturbances promptly, since corticosteroids can cause cataracts and glaucoma.

✔ Limit consumption of alcohol, caffeine, and aspirin to minimize gastric irritation caused by corticosteroids.

✔ Report any unexplained changes in mood as well as physical symptoms such as abdominal pain, bone pain, tiredness, easy bruising, and tarry stools.

✔ Minimize any changes in appearance with cosmetics and be assured that these changes will disappear at the end of therapy.

✔ Never stop taking the drug abruptly; rather, decrease the dosage gradually.

      f) Vaccines, toxoids: decreased response to vaccines and toxoids; heightened replication of attenuated virus, increasing risk of infection

      g) Estrogen: increased corticosteroid effects

      h) Cholestyramine: decreased corticosteroid absorption

      i) Isoniazid: reduced isoniazid effectiveness, increased corticosteroid effects

      j) Antihypertensives: antagonism of antihypertensive effects

B. Mineralocorticoids
   1. Examples: desoxycorticosterone pivalate (Percorten Pivalate), fludrocortisone (Florinef)
   2. Use/mechanism of action: treat adrenocortical insufficiency and inflammatory and immune reactions by affecting electrolyte and water balance
   3. Adverse effects
      a) Desoxycorticosterone: edema, hypertension, congestive heart failure, hypernatremia, hypokalemia, hypocalcemia
      b) Fludrocortisone: same as glucocorticoids (see section III,A,3,a–g in this chapter)
   4. Contraindications: heart disease, known hypersensitivity
   5. Precautions: Addison's disease, peptic ulcers, renal disease, osteoporosis, diabetes
   6. Drug interactions: same as III,A,6 in this chapter

C. Nursing diagnoses
   1. Potential for infection related to immunosuppression
   2. Body image disturbance related to hirsutism or altered fat distribution
   3. Fluid volume excess related to sodium and water retention
   4. Pain related to inflammatory disorder
   5. Altered thought process related to CNS side effects
   6. Impaired skin integrity related to dermatologic side effects
   7. Impaired physical mobility related to health disorder

D. Nursing implementation factors
 1. Administration procedures: Refrain from withdrawing glucocorticoids abruptly; gradually decrease dosage.
 2. Daily monitoring and measurements
    a) Monitor client for subtle signs of infection, such as increased white blood cell count (WBC).
    b) Take special precautions to avoid contamination of wounds, catheters, and tubes.
    c) Monitor serum glucose level, body weight, blood pressure, CBC, and electrolyte balance.
    d) Monitor client's blood pressure.
    e) Monitor fluid balance.
    f) Monitor client for changes in mood, particularly depression.
 3. Points for client teaching
    a) Warn client taking corticosteroids for more than 1 week not to stop drug abruptly.
    b) Tell client that corticosteroids can cause mood swings.
    c) Instruct client taking corticosteroids to report sore throat, cold, or other infection that lingers without improvement.
    d) Explain to client the importance of periodic evaluation of serum electrolyte levels and blood pressure.
    e) Advise client to reduce salt intake, monitor daily weight, and report signs of peripheral edema.

E. Nursing evaluations
 1. Client's inflammation and pain are decreased.
 2. Client shows no signs of infection.
 3. Client adapts to body image changes during glucocorticoid therapy.
 4. Client maintains normal hydration and fluid balance.
 5. Client's emotional state is stabilized.
 6. Client's skin integrity is maintained.
 7. Client experiences improved physical mobility.

See text pages
_____

IV. **Antidiabetic therapy**

A. Insulin
 1. Examples
    a) Rapid-acting insulin: Beef Regular Iletin II, Humulin R, Novolin R, Pork Regular Iletin II, Regular (Concentrated) Iletin II, Velosulin
    b) Prompt insulin zinc suspension (semilente): Semilente Iletin I, Semilente Purified Pork
    c) Intermediate-acting insulin (isophane insulin suspension, neutral protamine Hagedorn insulin [NPH]): Beef NPH Iletin II, Humulin N, Insulatard Human, Novolin N, NPH Insulin

      d) Insulin zinc suspension (lente): Humulin L, Lente Iletin I, Novolin L

      e) Long-acting insulin (protamine zinc suspension [PZI]): Protamine, Zinc & Iletin II (Beef)

      f) Extended insulin zinc suspension (ultralente): Ultralente Iletin I, Ultralente Purified Beef

      g) Insulin mixture (isophane insulin suspension with insulin injection): Mixtard, Novolin 70/30

2. Use/mechanism of action: treat type I diabetes mellitus (insulin-dependent diabetes mellitus [IDDM]); occasionally treat type II diabetes mellitus (noninsulin-dependent diabetes mellitus [NIDDM]) by facilitating glucose uptake, storage, and metabolism

3. Adverse effects: dose-related hypoglycemia (tachycardia, arrhythmias, headache, visual disturbances, diaphoresis, shakiness, apprehension, confusion, drowsiness, unconsciousness); hyperinsulinism resulting in rebound hyperglycemia (Somogyi effect) and insulin resistance; lipoatrophy and lipohypertrophy at injection site

4. Contraindications: hypoglycemia, hypersensitivity to particular insulin

5. Precautions: renal or hepatic dysfunction, pregnancy

6. Drug interactions

      a) Alcohol, anabolic steroids, salicylates, MAO (monoamine oxidase) inhibitors: hypoglycemia, reduced insulin dose

      b) Corticosteroids, sympathomimetics, thiazide-type diuretics: hyperglycemia, increased insulin dose

      c) Beta-blockers: masked hypoglycemia and delayed recovery from hypoglycemia

B. Oral hypoglycemic agents

1. Examples (sulfonylureas): acetohexamide (Dymelor), chlorpropamide (Glucamide), tolazamide (Tolinase), tolbutamide (Orinase), glipizide (Glucotrol), glyburide (Diabeta)

2. Use/mechanism of action: treat type II diabetes mellitus by stimulating the pancreas to release insulin

3. Adverse effects: dose-related hypoglycemia (tachycardia, arrhythmias, headache, visual disturbances, diaphoresis, shakiness, apprehension, confusion, drowsiness, unconsciousness)

4. Contraindications: pregnancy, lactation, diabetic ketoacidosis, known hypersensitivity

5. Precautions: renal or hepatic dysfunction

6. Drug interactions

      a) Alcohol: hypoglycemia or hyperglycemia

      b) Anabolic steroids, chloramphenicol, clofibrate, gemfibrozil, MAO inhibitors, phenylbutazone, salicylates, sulfonamides: hypoglycemia

      c) Corticosteroids, rifampin, sympathomimetics, thiazide-type diuretics: hyperglycemia

      d) Beta-blockers: modification of signs of hypoglycemia; masking of tachycardia and tremor; increased sweating

C. Nursing diagnoses

1. Altered health maintenance related to diabetes mellitus

2. Impaired skin integrity related to vascular pathology

        3. Altered nutrition, more (or less) than body requirements, related to medical condition

        4. High risk for fluid volume deficit related to adverse GI effects

        5. Potential for injury related to neuropathy

D. Nursing implementation factors

    1. Administration procedures

        a) Keep glucose or glucagon at hand to treat hypoglycemia reaction.

        b) Measure insulin carefully in appropriately gauged syringes (e.g., U-40, U-100).

        c) Avoid shaking insulin before measuring.

        d) Do not administer insulin that contains particles.

    2. Daily monitoring and measurements

        a) Monitor vital signs.

        b) Measure blood glucose level.

        c) Monitor fluid intake and output.

        d) Check body weight.

    3. Points for client teaching

        a) Instruct client with diabetes to recognize the symptoms of hypoglycemia and hyperglycemia (see Client Teaching Checklist, "Hypoglycemia and Hyperglycemia").

        b) Teach client how to store and measure insulin properly.

        c) Caution client not to change manufacturer, type, purity, or dosage of insulin unless instructed to do so by physician.

        d) Show client how to monitor blood glucose level and urine acetone levels.

        e) Provide guidance about appropriate diet and exercise regimens.

E. Nursing evaluations

    1. Client achieves therapeutic effect with no evidence of insulin side effects.

    2. Client monitors blood glucose and avoids hypoglycemia by having complex carbohydrate snack when level drops.

    3. Client maintains skin integrity.

    4. Client's food consumption is within normal limits.

    5. Client maintains normal hydration.

    6. Client is careful to avoid injury and checks extremities for signs of skin breakdown.

See text pages

_____

V. Pituitary hormones

A. Anterior pituitary agents

    1. Examples: corticotropin (ACTH), somatrem (Protropin)

    2. Use/mechanism of action: treat adrenal insufficiency, acute multiple sclerosis, myasthenia gravis, collagen diseases, diabetes insipidus; rheumatoid arthritis (corticotropin); and pituitary dwarfism

(somatrem) by binding with plasma membrane receptors to activate enzymes affecting metabolic rate in target organs

3. Adverse effects: dizziness, seizures, euphoria, insomnia, hallucinations, depression, psychosis, glaucoma, cataracts, impaired wound healing, impaired growth in children, edema, thrombophlebitis, arrhythmias, increased appetite, oral candidiasis, hyperglycemia

4. Contraindications: adrenocortical hyperfunction, known hypersensitivity

5. Precautions: tuberculosis, diabetes mellitus, renal impairment

6. Drug interactions

   a) Corticotropin and immunosuppressants: neurologic complications

   b) Corticotropin and salicylates: decreased salicylate levels

   c) Corticotropin with barbiturates, phenytoin, rifampin: decreased corticotropin effects

   d) Somatrem and corticosteroids: diminished growth response, glycosuria

B. Posterior pituitary agents

   1. Examples (synthetic antidiuretic hormone [ADH]): desmopressin (DDAVP), vasopressin (Pitressin)

   2. Use/mechanism of action: treat adrenal insufficiency and diabetes insipidus by regulating fluid balance, increasing water reabsorption in kidneys, and causing peripheral vasoconstriction

   3. Adverse effects: hypertension, angina, myocardial infarction, dizziness, light-headedness, trembling, headaches, drowsiness, confusion, seizures, coma, nausea, vomiting, abdominal cramps, diarrhea, flatus, hyponatremia, skin blanching, diaphoresis, water intoxication

   4. Contraindications: von Willebrand's disease, known hypersensitivity

   5. Precautions: cardiovascular disease, fluid overload, asthma

   6. Drug interactions

      a) Alcohol, demeclocycline, lithium: decreased ADH activity

  b) Chlorpropamide, clofibrate, carbamazepine, cyclophosphamide: increased ADH activity

  c) Barbiturate, cyclopropane anesthetics: coronary insufficiency, cardiac arrhythmia

C. Nursing diagnoses
 1. Anxiety related to medical condition
 2. Fluid volume excess or deficit related to sodium and water retention
 3. Altered oral mucous membranes related to fluid deficit

D. Nursing implementation factors
 1. Administration procedures
  a) Perform hypersensitivity skin test before administration.
  b) Keep epinephrine at hand for treatment of allergic reaction.
  c) Avoid discontinuing corticotropin administration abruptly.
  d) Match corticotropin solution type with method of administration: intravenous (IV) for aqueous solution, intramuscular (IM) or subcutaneous (SC) for suspension or gelatin.
 2. Daily monitoring and measurements
  a) Assess client's cardiovascular function regularly during ADH therapy.
  b) Monitor client's fluid intake and output during ADH therapy.
  c) Monitor client for urticaria, tachycardia, pruritus, and other signs of hypersensitivity.
  d) Watch for poor wound healing during corticotropin therapy.
 3. Points for client teaching
  a) Teach client how to monitor fluid intake and output while receiving ADH therapy.
  b) Tell client to report hives, rash, or other signs of hypersensitivity.

E. Nursing evaluations
 1. Client's medical condition is improved.
 2. Client achieves normal fluid balance.
 3. Client recognizes the importance of measuring and recording fluid intake and output.
 4. Client's oral mucous membranes remain intact.

VI. Male and female hormonal agents

See text pages
_____

A. Androgens
 1. Examples: testosterone (Testoject, DEPO-Testosterone, Andryl 200, Testex); danazol (Danocrine); fluoxymesterone (Halotestin)
 2. Use/mechanism of action: treat hypogonadism in males and treat breast cancer and endometriosis in females (danazol) by binding to androgen receptors in skeletal muscle, prostate, bone marrow, and other target organs, stimulating development and protein synthesis

3. Adverse effects: elevated serum cholesterol and serum calcium, sodium, and water retention (edema)
   a) In females: masculinization, menstrual irregularity, increased libido, mood swings
   b) In males: gynecomastia in adolescents, prostate enlargement, priapism, increased libido, oligospermia
   c) In children: premature growth plate closure, early development of male secondary sex characteristics
4. Contraindications: pregnancy, lactation, prostate cancer, breast cancer in males, liver or heart disease
5. Precautions: delayed puberty in boys
6. Drug interactions: bleeding with oral anticoagulants; edema with corticosteroids and high-sodium foods

B. Anabolic steroids
   1. Examples: ethylestrenol (Maxibolin), nandrolone (Durabolin), oxandrolone (Anavar), oxymetholone (Anadrol-50), testolactone (Teslac)
   2. Use/mechanism of action: treat osteoporosis, anemia, debilitation by increasing muscle mass and reducing catabolism and urinary elimination of nitrogen and electrolytes
   3. Adverse effects: same as VI,A,3 in this chapter
   4. Contraindications: pregnancy, lactation, prostate cancer, breast cancer in males, liver or heart disease
   5. Precautions: delayed puberty in boys
   6. Drug interactions: bleeding with oral anticoagulants; edema with corticosteroids and high-sodium foods

C. Estrogens and progestins
   1. Examples: conjugated estrogens (Estrocon, Premarin); diethylstilbestrol (DES); esterified estrogens (Estratab); estradiol (Estrace); estrone (Bestrone)
   2. Use/mechanism of action: treat estrogen deficiencies and prostate cancer; serve as contraception or estrogen replacement after menopause by promoting growth and development of female reproductive system and sharing pharmacologic properties of natural female sex hormone progesterone, which prepares endometrium for pregnancy and breasts for lactation
   3. Adverse effects
      a) Estrogens: long-term increased risk of endometrial cancer and gallbladder disease, mild hypertension, decreased glucose tolerance, altered menstrual flow, breast tenderness, mood changes, migraine headaches
      b) Progestins: altered menstrual flow, breast tenderness, breakthrough bleeding, mood changes, migraine headaches, increased risk of thrombophlebitis, pulmonary embolism, cerebral embolism (especially if female client smokes)
   4. Contraindications: pregnancy, thrombophlebitis, thromboembolic disorder, abnormal uterine bleeding, estrogen-dependent cancer of breast or reproductive organs

    5. Precautions: depression, metabolic bone disease, gallbladder disease, diabetes mellitus, amenorrhea, cardiac or renal impairment

    6. Drug interactions

        a) Estrogen with rifampin, barbiturates, carbamazepine, phenytoin, primidone: decreased estrogen effects

        b) Progestin with rifampin: increased progestin excretion

D. Nursing diagnoses

    1. Impaired tissue integrity related to metastatic disease

    2. Body image disturbance related to delayed development of secondary sex characteristics

    3. Fatigue related to anemia

    4. Pain related to endometriosis

E. Nursing implementation factors

    1. Administration procedures

        a) Mix estrogen or progestin prior to IM administration by rolling vial between the palms; administer deeply into large muscle.

        b) Perform complete physical and nutrition examination before initiating androgen/anabolic steroid therapy and obtain baseline values for CBC, serum cholesterol, serum calcium, and hepatic and cardiac function.

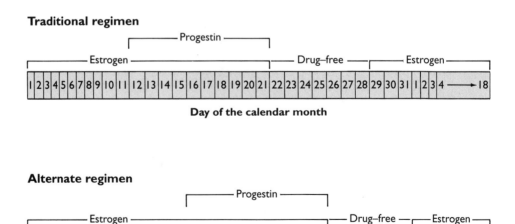

Figure 8–2
Calendar for Estrogen Regimens

2. Daily monitoring and measurements
   a) Measure body weight and fluid intake and output.
   b) Monitor blood pressure in client receiving estrogen/progestin.
   c) Watch client taking androgen/anabolic steroid for signs of hepatotoxicity.
   d) Monitor client taking androgen/anabolic steroid for signs of hypercalcemia, such as muscle weakness and bone pain; also be alert for arrhythmias if client is at risk because of bone cancer or parathyroid hormone oversecretion.
3. Points for client teaching
   a) Warn client against sharing androgenic or anabolic drug with others or using it for its body-building or aphrodisiac effects.
   b) Caution female client of childbearing age to use contraception if receiving progestin because that agent can cause fetal damage.
   c) Tell client taking estrogen/progestin that follow-up examinations are essential to detect diseases for which risk is increased, such as cancer.
   d) Teach client taking estrogen/progestin how to perform breast self-examination.

F. Nursing evaluations
   1. Client experiences decreased metastatic activity.
   2. Client's androgen deficiency is corrected.
   3. Client regains normal energy level as signs and symptoms of anemia are resolved.
   4. Client experiences reduced pain associated with menstrual cycle.

VII. Drugs affecting labor and lactation

See text pages

A. Uterine-stimulating agents
   1. Examples
      a) Oxytocin (Pitocin)
      b) Prostaglandins: carboprost (Prostin/15M), dinoprostone (Prostin E$_2$)
      c) Ergot alkaloids: ergonovine maleate (Ergotrate Maleate), methylergonovine maleate (Methergine)
   2. Use/mechanism of action: facilitate labor, induce abortion in second trimester, assist postdelivery, or treat involution of uterus by stimulating smooth muscle of uterus, causing contractions
   3. Adverse effects
      a) Oxytocin: nausea, vomiting, premature ventricular contractions, fetal bradycardia, dysrhythmias, neonatal jaundice (all occasional)
      b) Prostaglandins: nausea, vomiting, diarrhea, coughing, pain, fever, hypersensitivity
      c) Ergot alkaloids: nausea, vomiting, chest pain
   4. Contraindications
      a) Oxytocin: cord prolapse, fetal distress, hypertonic uterine patterns, preeclampsia, toxemia

        b) Prostaglandins: pelvic inflammatory disease, known hypersensitivity

        c) Ergot alkaloids: ergot hypersensitivity

    5. Precautions

        a) Oxytocin: history of trauma or major surgery to cervix or uterus, invasive cervical carcinoma, prematurity, fetal malposition

        b) Prostaglandins: cervical lacerations, uterine rupture

        c) Ergot alkaloids: coronary artery disease, hypertension, preeclampsia, hepatic or renal impairment, sepsis

    6. Drug interactions

        a) Oxytocin and prostaglandins: enhanced effects

        b) Prostaglandins and alcohol: antagonism of dinoprostone

        c) Ergot alkaloids and dopamine or vasoconstrictors: peripheral vasoconstriction with possible cyanosis and necrosis (see Nurse Alert, "Ergotamine Toxicity," in Chapter 3)

B. Uterine-inhibiting (tocolytic) agents

    1. Examples: ritodrine (Yutopar), terbutaline (Brethine)

    2. Use/mechanism of action: treat preterm labor by relaxing smooth muscle of uterus ($beta_2$-adrenergic agonists)

    3. Adverse effects: tremors, nausea, vomiting, headaches, tachycardia

    4. Contraindications: cardiac disease, hyperthyroidism, eclampsia, pulmonary hypertension, intrauterine infection, hemorrhage

    5. Precautions: diabetes, preeclampsia

    6. Drug interactions

        a) Long-acting corticosteroids (beclomethasone, dexamethasone, paramethasone): pulmonary edema, death

        b) Beta-blockers: mutual antagonism of effects

C. Lactation suppressants

    1. Examples: bromocriptine (Parlodel)

    2. Use/mechanism of action: stop milk production by decreasing serum prolactin levels

    3. Adverse effects: drowsiness, headache, nausea, hypotension

    4. Contraindications: uncontrolled hypertension, toxemia of pregnancy

    5. Precautions: hepatic impairment, psychiatric disorders

    6. Drug interactions: decreased effectiveness when administered with phenothiazines

D. Nursing diagnoses

    1. Pain related to breast engorgement

    2. Potential for injury related to postpartum bleeding

    3. Anxiety related to labor and delivery

    4. Potential fluid volume deficit related to vomiting caused by uterine motility agent

E. Nursing implementation factors
   1. Administration procedures
      a) Premedicate client with antiemetic to reduce vomiting and nausea.
      b) Observe client for hypersensitivity reactions after administration.
      c) Administer carboprost IM in deep muscle mass.
      d) Insert dinoprostone high into vagina and keep client supine for at least 10 minutes.
      e) Monitor uterine motility and fetal heart rate continuously during tocolytic agent administration.
   2. Daily monitoring and measurements
      a) Monitor vital signs, particularly blood pressure and temperature.
      b) Monitor client receiving tocolytic agent for chest tightness, chest pain, palpitations, and dyspnea.
      c) Monitor serum potassium and blood and urine glucose levels during therapy with tocolytic agent.
      d) Monitor neonate whose mother has received tocolytic therapy for increased heart rate, hypotension, and hypocalcemia.
   3. Points for client teaching
      a) Tell client to notify nurse or physician immediately if she experiences GI distress, difficult breathing, chest pain, or other adverse reactions.
      b) Let client know that it is a normal procedure to monitor vital signs throughout therapy.
      c) Provide emotional support for client terminating pregnancy or experiencing preterm labor and refer her to a support group if needed.

F. Nursing evaluations
   1. Client experiences effective uterine contractions and vaginal delivery of infant.
   2. Client experiences absence of breast engorgement.
   3. Client experiences reduction in postpartum bleeding.
   4. Client's vomiting is controlled.
   5. Neonate has normal vital signs following mother's tocolytic therapy.

1. Mrs. Maggiore, who is 65 years old, has just been diagnosed with hypothyroidism. She is started on levothyroxine sodium (Synthroid) 75 mcg daily. She should take this medication:
   a. At midmorning.
   b. With dinner.
   c. At bedtime.
   d. In 3 doses, with meals.

2. After taking levothyroxine sodium for a week, Mrs. Maggiore complains of tremors, nervousness, insomnia, and heart palpitations. The nurse should:
   a. Teach Mrs. Maggiore a relaxation exercise to reduce these side effects.
   b. Reassure Mrs. Maggiore that these are temporary effects and will decrease with time.
   c. Consult the physician about dividing the dose so she can take smaller amounts 3 times daily.
   d. Consult the physician about decreasing the dose.

3. A client who has received radioactive iodine to treat thyroid cancer should be told to take which of the following precautions for the first week after the dose is administered?
   a. Restrict fluids to 1500 ml/day.
   b. Avoid close contact with small children.
   c. Use uniodized salt.
   d. Use separate bathroom facilities from the rest of the family.

4. The nursing diagnosis that best addresses side effects of etidronate disodium (Didronel) administered to treat Paget's disease is:
   a. Potential for injury related to decreased bone mineralization.
   b. Fluid volume excess related to altered electrolyte metabolism.
   c. Constipation related to slowed peristalsis.
   d. Impaired swallowing related to enlarged thyroid gland.

5. A beclomethasone (Vanceril) inhaler is prescribed for Aletha Winters to treat asthma. Mrs. Winters should be taught to:
   a. Use the inhaler whenever she notices dyspnea and wheezing.
   b. Brush her teeth and rinse with diluted mouthwash after each inhalation.
   c. Use the beclomethasone before her prescribed bronchodilator to enhance its effect.
   d. Store her inhaler in the refrigerator.

6. The client who is taking oral prednisone should be advised to increase dietary intake of:
   a. Sodium.
   b. Iron.
   c. Potassium.
   d. Zinc.

7. Long-term corticosteroid therapy can produce Cushing's syndrome. The client receiving such therapy should be monitored for:
   a. Hypotension.
   b. Hypertrophy of leg muscles.
   c. Jaundice.
   d. Increased facial hair.

8. Mrs. Sommers receives 26 units of NPH insulin at 7:00 A.M. She is most likely to experience hypoglycemia when the insulin peaks, which would be:
   a. Around 9:00 A.M.
   b. During the afternoon.
   c. At bedtime.
   d. During the night.

9. If Mrs. Sommers experiences hypoglycemia, which symptom is she likely to evidence?
   a. Nausea
   b. Bradycardia
   c. Tremors
   d. Flushing

10. Mrs. Sommers's blood sugar levels have been high at 7:00 A.M., prior to her daily dose of insulin. The physician suspects the Somogyi phenomenon. To test for this, blood sugar must be checked at:

    a. 11:00 A.M.
    b. 4:00 P.M.
    c. 8:00 P.M.
    d. 3:00 A.M.

11. To evaluate for therapeutic effectiveness of lypressin (Diapid) nasal spray, the nurse should check the client's:

    a. Breath sounds.
    b. Skin color and temperature.
    c. Urine specific gravity.
    d. Blood glucose.

12. Mrs. Gardner has severe fibrocystic disease. Danazol (Danocrine) 100 mg BID is prescribed. She should be warned to report which sign of toxicity?

    a. Breast enlargement
    b. Increased libido
    c. Heavy menstrual flow
    d. Urine retention

ANSWERS

1. **Correct answer is a.** Thyroid hormone should be taken early in the day to minimize adverse effects on sleep patterns.

   b and **c.** Taking the drug with dinner or at bedtime is too late in the day. Peak drug effects produce nervousness and insomnia.
   d. The dose need not be divided, nor is administration with food required. A dose at dinnertime could interfere with sleep.

2. **Correct answer is d.** These are symptoms of excessive drug effect. Because Mrs. Maggiore is elderly, the usual adult dose may be too much for her. An elderly client may have cardiovascular problems that can be exacerbated by thyroid hormones.

   a. Relaxation exercises may help her manage the symptoms until the level of hormone in her blood drops, but dosage reduction is necessary to alleviate the symptoms.
   b. Since the client is experiencing toxic symptoms, reassurance is not an adequate response.
   c. Dividing the dose would not reduce the symptoms, since the total dose is too large.

3. **Correct answer is b.** The thyroid remains radioactive for up to 7 days, until all radioactive iodine is excreted. Small children may be adversely affected by the amount of radioactivity that prolonged close contact would expose them to.

   a. The client should force fluids to facilitate excretion of the radioactive iodine.
   c. The use of radioactive iodine does not affect the client's need for iodine as a nutrient.
   d. The amount of radioactive material excreted in urine is very small. It is safe for the client and family members to share a bathroom.

4. **Correct answer is a.** Etidronate disodium suppresses bone mineralization in the portion of the skeleton not affected by Paget's disease. This increases the client's risk of fractures.

   b. Fluid volume deficit is usually a result of nausea, vomiting, or diarrhea.
   c. Diarrhea, not constipation, is the anticipated intestinal effect.
   d. Etidronate disodium does not affect the thyroid gland and therefore does not affect swallowing. Thyroid enlargement occurs with hypothyroid conditions.

5. **Correct answer is b.** Corticosteroids suppress the body's defenses against infection. If inhaled beclomethasone is allowed to remain in the mouth, oral candidiasis is likely to occur.

   a. Beclomethasone is not a bronchodilator and will not relieve an acute asthma attack. It should be taken on a regular schedule to maintain its prophylactic effect.
   c. When both beclomethasone and a bronchodilator are prescribed, the bronchodilator

should be used first to open the airways and allow beclomethasone to reach the lower airways.

d. There is no need to refrigerate beclomethasone. The inhaler should be stored at room temperature in a clean place.

6. **Correct answer is c.** Because corticosteroids increase renal excretion of potassium and calcium, dietary intake of both nutrients should be increased.

a. Corticosteroids cause sodium retention. Increasing sodium intake would worsen this effect.
b and **d.** Iron and zinc are not affected by corticosteroids.

7. **Correct answer is d.** Hirsutism is one sign of Cushing's syndrome.

a. Corticosteroids cause sodium and fluid retention, so increased blood pressure is a common side effect.
b. In Cushing's syndrome, the extremities atrophy and muscles weaken. Muscle enlargement is more likely to occur with androgens.
c. Jaundice is a sign of liver dysfunction, which is not associated with corticosteroids.

8. **Correct answer is b.** NPH, which is an intermediate-acting insulin, peaks between 6 and 12 hours after administration.

a. The onset of action for NPH insulin is 1–2 hours after administration. Hypoglycemia is not as likely at the onset of action, in the morning, as at its peak.
c and **d.** The peak effect of NPH insulin is past by early evening, so hypoglycemia is unlikely to occur at bedtime or during the night.

9. **Correct answer is c.** Nervousness and tremors are common signs of hypoglycemia.

a. Nausea is not a sign of hypoglycemia. Hunger would be more likely.

b. Tachycardia is a sign of hypoglycemia. Bradycardia would not occur.
d. When the client is hypoglycemic, the skin becomes cool, pale, and diaphoretic.

10. **Correct answer is d.** The Somogyi phenomenon occurs when insulin continues to be absorbed from the injection site during the night, when there is no glucose for it to act upon. The body compensates for the resulting hypoglycemia by releasing glucagon, norepinephrine, and corticosteroids, which raise blood glucose levels above normal.

a, b, and **c.** Since the hypoglycemic episode occurs during the night, 11:00 A.M., 4:00 P.M., and 8:00 P.M. would not be appropriate times for detecting it. Blood sugars drawn at these times are used to evaluate the effectiveness of meal schedule and timing of insulin dose in controlling blood sugar.

11. **Correct answer is c.** Lypressin is a synthetic antidiuretic hormone (ADH) analogue used to treat diabetes insipidus. If treatment is effective, urine specific gravity will rise.

a. Since lypressin is not used to treat respiratory problems, breath sounds would not provide useful information.
b. Lypressin is not used for circulatory disorders, so skin color and temperature are not relevant.
d. Diabetes insipidus does not affect blood glucose levels, so blood glucose would not be useful in monitoring for therapeutic effect.

12. **Correct answer is b.** Masculinizing effects, such as increased libido, may be signs of toxicity and should be reported.

a. Breast enlargement occurs with female hormones, not with danazol.
c. Menstrual flow is more likely to decrease or menses may become irregular with danazol.
d. Changes in urinary output seldom occur with androgenic hormones.

9

Drugs for Treating Infection and Inflammation

OVERVIEW

I. Antibiotics
- A. Examples
- B. Use/mechanism of action
- C. Adverse effects
- D. Contraindications
- E. Precautions
- F. Drug interactions
- G. Nursing diagnoses
- H. Nursing implementation factors
- I. Nursing evaluations

II. Antiviral agents
- A. Examples
- B. Use/mechanism of action
- C. Adverse effects
- D. Contraindications
- E. Precautions
- F. Drug interactions
- G. Nursing diagnoses
- H. Nursing implementation factors
- I. Nursing evaluations

III. Antifungal agents
- A. Examples
- B. Use/mechanism of action
- C. Adverse effects
- D. Contraindications
- E. Precautions
- F. Drug interactions
- G. Nursing diagnoses
- H. Nursing implementation factors
- I. Nursing evaluations

IV. Antiparasitic agents
- A. Antimalarial agents
- B. Antiamebiasis agents
- C. Nursing diagnoses
- D. Nursing implementation factors
- E. Nursing evaluations

V. Anthelmintic agents
- A. Examples
- B. Use/mechanism of action
- C. Adverse effects
- D. Contraindications
- E. Precautions
- F. Drug interactions
- G. Nursing diagnoses
- H. Nursing implementation factors
- I. Nursing evaluations

VI. Antitubercular agents
- A. Examples
- B. Use/mechanism of action
- C. Adverse effects
- D. Contraindications
- E. Precautions
- F. Drug interactions
- G. Nursing diagnoses
- H. Nursing implementation factors
- I. Nursing evaluations

I. Antibiotics	II. Antiviral agents	III. Antifungal agents	IV. Antiparasitic agents	V. Anthelmintic agents

1. The nurse should remember that accurate culture and sensitivity results will be achieved only if blood, pus, and sputum specimens are obtained before the start of antimicrobial therapy.
2. The nurse should be aware that many clients stop taking an antibiotic before the full course of treatment is complete, and the nurse therefore should stress the importance, including rationale, of using all medication.
3. The nurse should question clients to determine whether they have been taking an antibiotic left over from a previous illness or obtained from an acquaintance; under those circumstances, culture results will be invalid.

GLOSSARY

aerobe—an organism that requires oxygen to live and grow

anaerobe—an organism that lives and grows without oxygen

bactericidal agent—an agent that kills bacteria

bacteriostatic agent—an agent that inhibits the growth or multiplication of bacteria

beta-lactam antibiotic—a group of antibiotics that prevent the cross-linking of peptidoglycan, leading to the formation of defective bacterial cell walls; members include penicillins, cephalosporins, carbapenems, and monobactams

beta-lactamase enzyme—one of a group of bacterial enzymes that destroy beta-lactam antibiotics

cestode—a tapeworm, which consists of a head and segments; adults live in the alimentary tract and related ducts of vertebrates; larvae live in a variety of organs and tissues

gram-negative bacteria—organisms that lose their stain in Gram's method of staining and have cell wall surfaces that are more chemically complex than those of gram-positive bacteria

gram-positive bacteria—organisms that retain their stain in Gram's method of staining and have cell wall surfaces that are composed of peptidoglycan and teichoic acid

nematode—a roundworm, belonging to the class of helminths

penicillinase—a bacterial enzyme that inactivates penicillin

trematode—a fluke, which belongs to the phylum *Platyhelminthes*

ENHANCED OUTLINE

See text pages

I. Antibiotics

A. Examples

    1. Penicillins: penicillin G, penicillin V (natural penicillins); methicillin (Staphcillin), oxacillin (Prostaphlin) (penicillinase-resistant penicillins);

amoxicillin (Omnipen), carbenicillin (Geopen), piperacillin (Pipracil), ticarcillin (Ticar) (extended spectrum penicillins)

2. Cephalosporins: cefadroxil (Duricef), cefazolin (Ancef), cephalexin monohydrate (Keflex) (first-generation cephalosporins); cefaclor (Ceclor), cefamandole (Mandol), cefoxitin (Mefoxin), cefuroxime axetil (Ceftin) (second-generation cephalosporins); cefixime (Suprax), cefotaxime (Claforan), cefotetan (Cefotan), ceftazidime (Fortaz), ceftriaxone (Rocephin) (third-generation cephalosporins)

3. Aminoglycosides: amikacin (Amikin), gentamicin (Garamycin), kanamycin (Kantrex), neomycin (Neobiotic), netilmicin (Netromycin), streptomycin, tobramycin (Nebcin)

4. Tetracyclines: chlortetracycline (Aureomycin), oxytetracycline (Terramycin), tetracycline (Achromycin) (short-acting); demeclocycline (Declomycin), methacycline (Rondomycin) (intermediate-acting); doxycycline (Vibramycin), minocycline (Minocin) (long-acting)

5. Urinary tract drugs: ciprofloxacin (Cipro), norfloxacin (Noroxin), ofloxacin (Floxin) (quinolones); co-trimoxazole (Bactrim), sulfadiazine (Microsulfon), sulfamethoxazole (Gantanol), sulfisoxazole (Gantrisin) (sulfonamides); nitrofurantoin (Furadantin, Macrodantin)

6. Miscellaneous antibiotics: chloramphenicol (Chloromycetin), erythromycin (Erythrocin), lincomycin (Lincocin), clindamycin (Cleocin), imipenem-cilastatin (Primaxin), vancomycin (Vancocin), aztreonam (Azactam)

B. Use/mechanism of action: kill bacteria (bactericidal antibiotics) or limit their growth (bacteriostatic antibiotics) by either interfering with cell wall synthesis of the microorganism or interfering with intracellular metabolism; broad-spectrum agents effective against many different microorganisms, narrow-spectrum effective against a few microorganisms

C. Adverse effects

1. General: hypersensitivity reactions (most common), gastrointestinal (GI) distress, hepatotoxicity, nephrotoxicity

2. Particular

a) Penicillins: vaginitis, hemolytic anemia and platelet dysfunction (at high doses)

b) Cephalosporins: pain at intramuscular (IM) site, bleeding, thrombophlebitis (with intravenous [IV] cephalothin)

c) Aminoglycosides: ototoxicity

d) Tetracyclines: superinfection, tooth-enamel discoloration in children, photosensitivity; vestibular disturbances, such as dizziness

e) Urinary tract drugs

(1) Quinolones: crystalluria, dry mouth, photosensitivity, blurred or double vision, dizziness, light-headedness, drowsiness, headache, seizures, hallucinations, depression

(2) Sulfonamides: crystalluria and tubular deposits of sulfonamide crystals at high doses; nausea, vomiting, diarrhea; fever

(3) Nitrofurantoin: GI upset, peripheral neuropathy appearing as paresthesia in legs, possible precipitation of asthma attacks or

acute pneumonitis in elderly, urine discoloration, leukopenia or granulocytopenia (rare)

    f) Miscellaneous antibiotics

        (1) Chloramphenicol: bone marrow suppression (reversible), aplastic anemia (usually irreversible), gray syndrome in infants (see Nurse Alert, "Gray Syndrome")

        (2) Erythromycin: cholestatic hepatitis, reversible hearing loss (rare)

        (3) Lincomycin and clindamycin: pseudomembranous colitis (see Nurse Alert, "Pseudomembranous Colitis")

        (4) Imipenem-cilastatin: phlebitis or thrombophlebitis at infusion site, seizures in elderly or clients with seizure disorder (occasional)

        (5) Vancomycin: ototoxicity; mild hematuria, proteinuria, casts, azotemia; hypotension with rapid IV administration

        (6) Aztreonam: numbness of tongue, oral ulceration; transient eosinophilia, leukopenia, neutropenia; thrombophlebitis; hypotension; adverse central nervous system (CNS) effects such as seizures, dizziness, headache (occasional)

D. Contraindications

    1. Pregnancy: all agents except penicillins, cephalosporins, and chloramphenicol

    2. Lactation: tetracyclines, quinolones, lincomycin, clindamycin, sulfonamides

    3. Neonates: tetracyclines, nitrofurantoin

    4. Infancy to age 8: tetracyclines

    5. Renal disease: nitrofurantoin

    6. Hearing impairment: vancomycin

! NURSE *ALERT* !

Gray Syndrome

High chloramphenicol serum concentrations can cause gray syndrome, a rare but potentially fatal complication. It is most common in neonates and can be recognized by:

- Abdominal distention
- Vomiting
- Anorexia
- Tachypnea
- Cyanosis
- Green stools
- Lethargy
- Gray, ashen skin color

Gray syndrome may progress to circulatory collapse and death.

Pseudomembranous Colitis

Clindamycin and lincomycin can produce pseudomembranous colitis, a rare but potentially fatal condition caused by toxins secreted by *Clostridium difficile,* a bacterial species that overgrows in the presence of these antibiotics. The initial drug must be discontinued promptly and follow-up treatment begun with vancomycin or metronidazole. Signs and symptoms of pseudomembranous colitis include:
- Severe diarrhea
- Abdominal pain
- Fever
- Mucus and blood in stools

E. Precautions: renal or hepatic impairment (unless contraindicated)
   1. Neonates: chloramphenicol
   2. Seizure disorder: quinolones, imipenem-cilastatin
   3. Gastrointestinal disease (especially colitis): cephalosporins, lincomycin, gentamicin
   4. Allergies or asthma: penicillins, sulfonamides, lincomycin, clindamycin
   5. Hypersensitivity to penicillin: imipenem-cilastatin, aztreonam
   6. Hypersensitivity to cephalosporins: aztreonam
   7. Other precautions: mononucleosis, hemorrhagic disorder, or electrolyte imbalance with penicillins; advanced age or neuromuscular disease with aminoglycosides

F. Drug interactions
   1. Penicillins
      a) Methotrexate: interference with renal tubular secretion of methotrexate
      b) Probenecid: increased plasma penicillin concentration
      c) Tetracyclines or chloramphenicol: impaired bactericidal action of penicillins
      d) Neomycin: decreased absorption of penicillin V
      e) Oral contraceptives: decreased contraceptive efficacy when taken with penicillin V or ampicillin
   2. Cephalosporins
      a) Alcohol: acute alcohol intolerance, accompanied by headache, nausea, flushing, dizziness, vomiting, and abdominal cramps, when taken with cefamandole, cefoperazone, and moxalactam
      b) Imipenem-cilastatin: cephalosporin antagonism
      c) Probenecid: increased effectiveness of cephalosporins because of reduced renal tubular secretion
   3. Aminoglycosides
      a) Antihistamines: masked ototoxicity
      b) Loop diuretics: increased ototoxicity
      c) Methoxyflurane: additive nephrotoxicity and neurotoxicity
      d) Neuromuscular blocking agents: increased blockades

Drugs for Treating Infection and Inflammation   165

e) Carbenicillin, ticarcillin, azlocillin, mezlocillin, piperacillin, gentamicin, tobramycin with amphotericin B, cephalosporins, acyclovir, cyclosporines: inactivation of aminoglycosides

4. Tetracyclines

   a) Aluminum and magnesium antacids: inhibition of GI absorption of tetracyclines
   b) Methoxyflurane: nephrotoxicity
   c) Penicillin: interference with effectiveness of penicillin if concurrently administered
   d) Iron salts, bismuth subsalicylate, zinc sulfate: decreased GI absorption of tetracyclines
   e) Barbiturates, carbamazepine, phenytoin: increased metabolism of doxycycline
   f) Oral contraceptives: altered GI flora, decreased contraception, breakthrough bleeding

5. Urinary tract drugs

   a) Quinolones
      (1) Probenecid: decreased ciprofloxacin absorption, decreased excretion of ciprofloxacin and norfloxacin
      (2) Theophylline: increased theophylline levels with all quinolones
      (3) Magnesium- and aluminum-containing antacids: decreased quinolone absorption
   b) Sulfonamides
      (1) Para-aminobenzoic acid: decreased antibacterial effects of sulfonamides
      (2) Sulfonylurea hypoglycemic agents: increased hypoglycemic effects when administered with sulfonamides
      (3) Methenamine: increased risk of crystalluria with sulfonamides
      (4) Co-trimoxazole with coumarin anticoagulants: increased anticoagulant effects
      (5) Co-trimoxazole with cyclosporine: additive nephrotoxicity
   c) Nitrofurantoin
      (1) Probenecid, sulfinpyrazone: reduced efficacy and increased risk of toxicity
      (2) Antacids: decreased or delayed nitrofurantoin absorption
      (3) Norfloxacin, nalidixic acid: reduced antibacterial activity

6. Miscellaneous antibiotics

   a) Chloramphenicol: inhibition of metabolism of oral hypoglycemic agents, phenytoins, and oral anticoagulants when taken with chloramphenicol, causing increased effects and increased risk of toxicity
   b) Erythromycin
      (1) Theophylline: increased theophylline levels, heightening the risk of toxicity

        (2) Vitamin B complex, vitamin C, cephalothin, tetracycline, heparin, chloramphenicol: incompatibility when combined in solution with erythromycin

    c) Lincomycin and clindamycin

        (1) Neuromuscular blocking agents: increased blockade when administered with lincomycin or clindamycin

        (2) Kaolin preparations: greatly reduced lincomycin absorption

        (3) Ampicillin, aminophylline, calcium gluconate, magnesium sulfate: incompatibility with clindamycin

    d) Imipenem-cilastatin

        (1) Probenecid: increased, prolonged serum levels of cilastatin (which is not antibacterial) and slightly increased imipenem level

        (2) Aminoglycosides: synergistic action against *Streptococcus faecalis,* lack of effectiveness against most *Pseudomonas aeruginosa* strains when administered with imipenem-cilastatin

        (3) Chloramphenicol: decreased effectiveness of imipenem-cilastatin against *Klebsiella pneumoniae*

    e) Vancomycin: additive toxicity of aminoglycosides, amphotericin B, cisplatin, bacitracin, polymyxin B and other nephrotoxic or ototoxic drugs when administered with vancomycin

    f) Aztreonam

        (1) Aminoglycosides and other beta-lactam antibiotics: synergistic or additive effects

        (2) Cefoxitin, imipenem-cilastatin: possible inactivation of aztreonam

        (3) Chloramphenicol: antagonism if administered within 2 hours of aztreonam

        (4) Clavulanic acid: synergistic or antagonistic effect with aztreonam, depending on infectious organism

G. Nursing diagnoses

  1. Fluid volume deficit related to vomiting and diarrhea

  2. Hyperthermia related to infection

  3. Potential for infection related to superinfection

  4. Diarrhea related to antibiotic administration

  5. Knowledge deficit related to purpose of prescribed antibiotic

  6. Sensory-perceptual alterations: auditory related to ototoxicity (aminoglycosides, vancomycin)

  7. Sensory-perceptual alterations: visual related to photosensitivity or blurred or double vision (urinary tract drugs)

  8. High risk for trauma related to seizures (quinolones and imipenem-cilastatin)

  9. Altered urinary elimination related to crystalluria and tubular deposits (sulfonamides)

 10. Impaired tissue integrity related to pseudomembranous colitis (lincomycin or clindamycin)

H. Nursing implementation factors (see Client Teaching Checklist, "Antibiotic Administration")

I. Antibiotics	II. Antiviral agents	III. Antifungal agents	IV. Antiparasitic agents	V. Anthelmintic agents

1. Administration procedures
   a) All antibiotics
      (1) Collect appropriate specimen for culture and sensitivity tests before the start of therapy.
      (2) Keep emergency equipment at hand in case of a hypersensitivity response.
      (3) Check client's history of allergies.
   b) Penicillins
      (1) Have emergency equipment and epinephrine at hand in case of anaphylactic shock.
      (2) Administer oral penicillin 1 hour before or 2 hours after meals.
      (3) Refrain from mixing penicillins and aminoglycosides in same syringe.
   c) Cephalosporins
      (1) Infuse IV cephalosporins over a 30-minute period.
      (2) Administer oral (PO) cephalosporins with food to reduce GI upset.
   d) Aminoglycosides: Administer an aminoglycoside and extended-spectrum penicillin or cephalosporin at least 2 hours apart when using combination therapy.
   e) Tetracyclines
      (1) Administer long-acting compounds with food to reduce GI upset.
      (2) Avoid administering tetracyclines, except for long-acting compounds, with milk or milk products.
   f) Urinary tract drugs
      (1) Increase fluid intake during therapy with a urinary tract drug.
      (2) Administer quinolones on an empty stomach.
      (3) Take safety precautions if client shows CNS adverse effects during quinolone therapy.
      (4) Reduce gastric upset by administering nitrofurantoin with food or milk.

✔ CLIENT TEACHING CHECKLIST ✔

Antibiotic Administration

Explanations to the client:

✔ Complete the full course of your therapy even if you are symptom-free.

✔ It is important to maintain adequate drug levels in the blood by taking medication exactly as prescribed and at evenly spaced intervals.

✔ Discontinue the drug and contact your physician or nurse immediately if you experience a rash, itching, hives, fever, chills, joint pain or swelling, or wheezing or difficulty in breathing.

g) Chloramphenicol: Monitor client's serum drug level, bearing in mind that toxic response can occur at levels of 40 mcg/ml and above.

h) Erythromycin

    (1) Refrain from mixing in same syringe with vitamin B complex, vitamin C, cephalothin, tetracycline, heparin, or chloramphenicol.

    (2) Reconstitute solutions in normal saline or 5% dextrose and administer within 4 hours of preparation.

    (3) Avoid administering with food.

    (4) Refrain from administering IM.

i) Lincomycin and clindamycin: Keep reconstituted clindamycin solution for up to 2 weeks but do not refrigerate.

j) Imipenem-cilastatin: Avoid mixing with other antibiotics in same syringe.

k) Vancomycin

    (1) Refrain from administering IM.

    (2) Administer IV slowly, over a 30–60 minute period, to prevent hypotension.

    (3) Administer vancomycin orally only for *Clostridium difficile*–induced pseudomembranous colitis and staphylococcal enterocolitis.

2. Daily monitoring and measurements

a) All antibiotics

    (1) Document clinical signs and symptoms of infection.

    (2) Monitor fluid intake and output.

    (3) Monitor peak and trough levels of drug.

    (4) Monitor client for signs and symptoms of superinfection, including diarrhea, oral thrush, and vaginal itching.

b) Penicillins

    (1) Observe client during first week of therapy for symptoms of serum sickness, including fever, urticaria, joint pain, and angioneurotic edema.

    (2) Monitor hemoglobin concentration and electrolytes.

c) Cephalosporins: Monitor client receiving cephalosporin for signs of nephrotoxicity, including increases in serum urea nitrogen and creatine levels, changes in urine output, water retention, and proteinuria.

d) Aminoglycosides

    (1) Monitor serum creatinine level.

    (2) Check for hearing loss regularly, particularly in elderly clients.

    (3) Observe client for signs of vestibular toxicity, including dizziness, nystagmus, vertigo, and/or ataxia.

e) Tetracyclines: Review blood urea nitrogen (BUN) and creatinine levels and results of liver function studies for abnormalities.

f) Urinary tract drugs

    (1) Monitor client taking quinolone for crystalluria, checking for blood in urine and lower back pain.

    (2) Observe client taking quinolone for adverse CNS effects.

    (3) Monitor urinary elimination pattern during sulfonamide therapy to confirm that daily output is 1500 ml or greater.

  (4) Question client receiving nitrofurantoin about numbness or tingling in legs.

 g) Chloramphenicol

  (1) Monitor clients receiving high doses for signs and symptoms of gray syndrome.

  (2) Check client's mouth regularly for stomatitis.

  (3) Observe client for anemia, infection or bleeding, and signs of aplastic anemia, which can occur after drug is stopped.

 h) Erythromycin

  (1) Check client for hearing loss.

  (2) Monitor client for hepatic dysfunction.

  (3) Observe client for signs and symptoms of cholestatic hepatitis, including nausea, vomiting, abdominal pain, jaundice, rash, leukocytosis, and eosinophilia.

 i) Lincomycin and clindamycin: Check client's mouth for signs of stomatitis.

 j) Imipenem-cilastatin: Watch liver study results for transient elevations in aspartate aminotransferase (AST), alanine aminotransferase (ALT), and lactate dehydrogenase (LDH).

 k) Vancomycin

  (1) Monitor serum creatinine if renal impairment is present or another nephrotoxic compound is also being administered.

  (2) Observe client for signs of ototoxicity, including tinnitus and hearing loss.

 l) Aztreonam

  (1) Check for mouth ulceration.

  (2) Take seizure precautions, such as keeping padded tongue blade at bedside.

3. Points for client teaching

 a) All antibiotics

  (1) Teach client the signs and symptoms of allergic reaction.

  (2) Instruct client when to take antibiotic.

 b) Penicillins: Instruct client to take penicillin 1 hour before or 2 hours after meals.

 c) Cephalosporins

  (1) Caution client with diabetes that cephalosporins can cause false-positive results on urine glucose tests.

  (2) Warn client against using alcohol while taking moxalactam, cefoperazone, cefamandole, or cefotetan.

 d) Aminoglycosides

  (1) Instruct client to contact nurse or physician immediately if he/she experiences an irregular heartbeat, difficulty in breathing, or hearing loss.

(2) Explain to client that blood tests are necessary during aminogly-coside therapy to gauge effectiveness and detect adverse effects.
- e) Tetracyclines
    (1) Tell client never to take drug with over-the-counter (OTC) products such as antacids and vitamins that contain calcium, magnesium, aluminum, or iron.
    (2) Instruct client to avoid direct sunlight and use a sunscreen (SPF 15+) if exposure is unavoidable.
    (3) Advise female clients taking birth control pills to use another method of contraception until 1 week after therapy is complete, as efficacy of birth control pills is decreased by tetracyclines.
- f) Urinary tract drugs
    (1) Suggest that client receiving quinolone use sugarless candy and ice chips to relieve dry mouth and increase fluid intake to avoid crystalluria.
    (2) Warn client taking quinolone that since dizziness or drowsiness may occur, he/she should avoid operating machinery until drug effects are known.
    (3) Advise client taking sulfonamide to avoid photosensitivity effects by avoiding unnecessary exposure to sunlight and to apply sunblock with an SPF of more than 15 prior to any exposure.
    (4) Instruct client to increase fluid intake while receiving sulfonamide therapy.
    (5) Explain to client that nitrofurantoin may cause harmless change in urine color.
    (6) Tell client receiving nitrofurantoin to contact physician immediately if he/she experiences hypersensitivity reaction or changed sensation in legs.
- g) Chloramphenicol
    (1) Tell client to report fever, sore throat, unexplained fatigue, or unusual bleeding or bruising.
    (2) Warn client that drug has an unpleasant taste.
    (3) Explain to client that blood tests during therapy are important.
- h) Erythromycin
    (1) Explain to client that liver function tests are important during long-term therapy.
    (2) Advise client to notify nurse or physician if hearing changes occur.
- i) Lincomycin and clindamycin
    (1) Warn client that IM injection may be painful and that any subsequent pain at injection site should be reported.
    (2) Describe to client the symptoms of pseudomembranous colitis and instruct him/her to report them immediately if they arise.
- j) Imipenem-cilastatin: Explain the need for laboratory studies during imipenem-cilastatin therapy.

         k) Vancomycin: Tell client to report tinnitus or hearing loss.

         l) Aztreonam: Teach client how to manage mouth ulcers.

I. Nursing evaluations

1. Client achieves good therapeutic response without evidence of allergic reaction.
2. An absence of bacterial growth is found on client's laboratory cultures.
3. Client experiences absence of signs and symptoms of infection, including pain, redness, swelling, and drainage.
4. Client's white blood cell count (WBC) and hemoglobin concentration are normal.
5. Client reports no tinnitus or hearing loss after aminoglycoside or vancomycin therapy.
6. Client voids urine normally with no evidence of drug crystallization after administration of urinary tract drug.
7. Client is free from seizure activity after therapy with a quinolone or with imipenem-cilastatin.

II. Antiviral agents

See text pages
_____

A. Examples: acyclovir (Zovirax), ganciclovir (Cytovene), vidarabine (Vira-A), amantadine (Symmetrel), ribavirin (Virazole), zidovudine (Retrovir)

B. Use/mechanism of action: treat viruses such as herpes simplex virus (HSV), influenza A and B, cytomegalovirus (CMV), and human immunodeficiency virus (HIV) by inhibiting virus-specific enzymes involved in DNA synthesis

C. Adverse effects

1. Acyclovir: local reactions at parenteral injection site; reversible renal impairment; headache and GI distress with oral drug
2. Ganciclovir: granulocytopenia, thrombocytopenia
3. Vidarabine: GI upset; CNS effects, including weakness, tremor, malaise, confusion, hallucinations
4. Amantadine: nausea, anorexia, nervousness, fatigue, depression, irritability
5. Ribavirin: worsening of symptoms in clients with respiratory infections (uncommon)
6. Zidovudine: anemia, granulocytopenia; headache and other CNS symptoms; GI upset

D. Contraindications: pregnancy (with ribavirin), lactation (with vidarabine and ribavirin), mechanical ventilation (with ribavirin)

E. Precautions

1. Acyclovir and ganciclovir: pregnancy, lactation, renal impairment
2. Vidarabine: pregnancy, CNS infection, renal or hepatic impairment

3. Amantadine: hepatic impairment, eczema, psychosis
4. Ribavirin: respiratory impairment, asthma
5. Zidovudine: pregnancy, renal or hepatic impairment

F. Drug interactions
   1. Acyclovir: increased risk of renal dysfunction with nephrotoxic agents
   2. Ganciclovir
      a) Probenecid: reduced elimination and increased serum concentration of ganciclovir
      b) Cytotoxic drugs (e.g., dapsone, pentamidine, flucytosine, vincristine, doxorubicin, trimethoprim, sulfamethoxazole): inhibition of normal cell replication in bone marrow, skin, GI tract; additive toxicity
      c) Imipenem-cilastatin: increased risk of seizures
      d) Zidovudine: granulocytopenia
   3. Vidarabine: vidarabine toxicity, including tremor, anemia, nausea, pruritus, and pain, with allopurinol
   4. Amantadine: enhanced anticholinergic effects with anticholinergics
   5. Ribavirin
      a) Cardiac glycoside: cardiac glycoside intoxication
      b) Zidovudine: increased hematologic adverse effects, possibly because of zidovudine antagonism
   6. Zidovudine
      a) Dapsone, pentamidine, flucytosine, vincristine, vinblastine, doxorubicin, interferon, ganciclovir: increased cytotoxic and nephrotoxic effects
      b) Probenecid, aspirin, acetaminophen, indomethacin, cimetidine, lorazepam: increased risk of toxicity from both agents
      c) Acyclovir: extreme drowsiness and lethargy

G. Nursing diagnoses
   1. Potential fluid volume deficit related to vomiting and diarrhea
   2. High risk of infection related to superinfection

H. Nursing implementation factors
   1. Administration procedures
      a) Administer IV acyclovir or ganciclovir slowly to avoid crystallization in renal tubules; use a vein with good flow and rotate IV sites regularly to avoid phlebitis.
      b) Administer only clear vidarabine solutions and use an in-line filter (0.45 micron or finer); do not exceed 450 mg of drug per liter of solution.
      c) Monitor client receiving ribavirin therapy for hypotension and signs of cardiac arrest and have emergency equipment at hand.
      d) Administer ribavirin only with the SPAG-2 aerosol generator.
   2. Daily monitoring and measurements
      a) Measure serum creatinine level during acyclovir or ganciclovir therapy.
      b) Monitor complete blood count (CBC) and neutrophil and platelet counts regularly during therapy with acyclovir, ganciclovir, and zidovudine.

        c) Observe client closely during ganciclovir therapy for signs of occult bleeding caused by thrombocytopenia.

        d) Measure fluid intake and output during vidarabine therapy for signs of fluid volume excess.

        e) Monitor client with history of congestive heart failure for signs of recurrence during amantadine therapy.

        f) Assess client's respiratory function hourly during ribavirin therapy.

    3. Points for client teaching

        a) Caution women of childbearing age to use birth control during ganciclovir therapy because of the drug's potential for mutagenic effects.

        b) Advise mother of infant not to breastfeed during ganciclovir therapy.

        c) Instruct client to take amantadine after meals.

        d) Suggest that client take amantadine well before bedtime if he/she experiences insomnia while taking it.

        e) Tell client receiving zidovudine the drug should be taken every 4 hours; client should set an alarm at night to wake up at proper time.

        f) Tell client taking zidovudine that the drug will not reduce the risk of transmitting the AIDS virus to others.

I. Nursing evaluations

    1. Client shows an absence of signs and symptoms of infection.

    2. There is an absence of viral growth on laboratory culture.

III. Antifungal agents

See text pages

A. Examples: amphotericin B (Fungizone), nystatin (Mycostatin), flucytosine (Ancobon), fluconazole (Diflucan), ketoconazole (Nizoral)

B. Use/mechanism of action: treat systemic and topical fungal infections by interfering with synthesis and functioning of fungal sterol, thereby inhibiting fungal growth

C. Adverse effects

    1. Amphotericin B: chills, fever, nausea, vomiting, anorexia, muscle and joint pain, abdominal pain, headache, weight loss at beginning of therapy; potentially quite toxic, causing nephrotoxicity and hypokalemia

    2. Nystatin: diarrhea, nausea, vomiting, abdominal pain (all rare)

    3. Flucytosine: bone marrow depression leading to anemia, leukopenia, thrombocytopenia at high serum levels; severe GI irritation; interference with normal renal functioning, leading to azotemia, elevation of BUN and serum creatinine, and crystalluria

4. Fluconazole: dizziness, headache, GI irritation, transient increases in AST, ALT, alkaline phosphatase, and bilirubin
5. Ketoconazole: nausea and vomiting; less commonly, CNS and skin effects, rashes, headache, dizziness, and insomnia

D. Contraindications
1. All antifungals: previous skin irritation with use, known hypersensitivity
2. Amphotericin B: lactation
3. Flucytosine: pregnancy, lactation
4. Ketoconazole: mild fungal infections of skin or nails (due to potential liver toxicity)

E. Precautions
1. Amphotericin B: pregnancy
2. Nystatin: pregnancy
3. Flucytosine: renal impairment, bone marrow depression, advanced age
4. Fluconazole: pregnancy, lactation, advanced age, childhood
5. Ketoconazole: impaired kidney or liver function

F. Drug interactions
1. Amphotericin B
   a) Aminoglycosides, cyclosporine, acyclovir: increased nephrotoxicity
   b) Corticosteroids, extended-spectrum penicillins, cardiac glycosides: increased hypokalemia
   c) Nondepolarizing skeletal muscle relaxants: increased relaxant effects
   d) Electrolytes: precipitation and inactivation of amphotericin B if mixed in same container
2. Nystatin: none significant
3. Flucytosine: none significant
4. Fluconazole
   a) Warfarin: increased prothrombin time
   b) Phenytoin, cyclosporine: increased levels of phenytoin and cyclosporine
   c) Rifampin: speeds up metabolism of fluconazole, reducing its efficacy
5. Ketoconazole
   a) Cimetidine, ranitidine, famotidine, antacids, anticholinergics: decreased absorption of ketoconazole
   b) Theophylline: decreased theophylline levels
   c) Other hepatotoxic drugs (e.g., aminoglycosides): increased hepatotoxicity
   d) Oral anticoagulants: increased anticoagulant effects

G. Nursing diagnoses
1. Potential for infection related to superinfection
2. Hyperthermia related to fever
3. Potential for altered urinary elimination related to nephrotoxicity
4. Potential for impaired tissue integrity related to phlebitis at IV administration site

H. Nursing implementation factors
1. Administration procedures
    a) Dilute amphotericin B with sterile water or a D_5W solution with a pH greater than 4.1, not an electrolyte solution.
    b) Infuse fluconazole at a rate of 200 mg/hour or less.
    c) Refrain from administering ketoconazole with antacids, anticholinergics, or other drugs that reduce gastric acidity.
2. Daily monitoring and measurements
    a) Monitor serum electrolytes during amphotericin B treatment.
    b) Measure BUN and serum creatinine levels during therapy with amphotericin B, flucytosine, or fluconazole.
    c) Assess hydration in client who experiences severe GI distress while being treated with nystatin or flucytosine.
    d) Monitor liver function tests during ketoconazole therapy.
    e) Monitor client's temperature during treatment with antifungal agent.
3. Points for client teaching
    a) Warn client that fever, chills, GI upset, and head, muscle, joint, and abdominal pain will probably occur at the start of amphotericin B treatment but should subside as therapy continues.
    b) Tell client with oral candidiasis to let nystatin tablet dissolve in mouth rather than chewing or swallowing it.
    c) Tell client receiving flucytosine to report sore throat, fever, unusual bruising, bleeding, fatigue, or weakness.

I. Nursing evaluations
1. Client has no signs or symptoms of fungal infection.
2. Client shows no evidence of adverse hematologic effects.
3. Client's BUN and serum creatinine remain normal, with no evidence of nephrotoxicity.
4. Client has no signs of phlebitis at IV site.
5. Client's temperature is normal.

IV. Antiparasitic agents

See text pages
_____

A. Antimalarial agents
1. Examples: chloroquine, hydroxychloroquine, mefloquine, primaquine, pyrimethamine, quinine
2. Use/mechanism of action: treat malaria by binding to and altering protozoal DNA, depleting folates, and reducing nucleic acid and protein production
3. Adverse effects: GI upset; cinchonism, a toxic syndrome marked by tinnitus, headache, vertigo, fever, light-headedness, and changes in vision (quinine)

4. Contraindications: pregnancy, blackwater fever, optic neuritis, psoriasis, porphyria, known hypersensitivity
5. Precautions: lactation, renal or hepatic impairment, severe allergies or asthma, seizure disorder
6. Drug interactions
   a) Chloroquine with magnesium-containing antacids: reduction of chloroquine absorption
   b) Hydroxychloroquine and digoxin: increased digoxin concentrations
   c) Mefloquine with beta-blockers, calcium channel blockers, quinine, quinidine: ECG abnormalities, cardiac arrest
   d) Primaquine and quinacrine: increased risk of primaquine toxicity
   e) Pyrimethamine and folic acid: inhibition of antimicrobial effect

B. Antiamebiasis agents
   1. Examples: emetine; furazolidone (Furoxone); iodoquinol (Diquinol, Moebiquin, Yodoxin); metronidazole (Flagyl, Metryl, Satric); paromomycin (Humatin); pentamidine (Pentam 300, NebuPent); quinacrine (Atabrine)
   2. Use/mechanism of action: treat acute intestinal amebiasis or acute amebic dysentery by poorly understood mechanism or by blocking of protein synthesis (emetine)
   3. Adverse effects: GI distress; cardiovascular effects (emetine); dose-related neurotoxicity (iodoquinol)
   4. Contraindications: first-trimester pregnancy, lactation, known hypersensitivity; cardiac or renal disease (emetine)
   5. Precautions: childhood, advanced age, hepatic disease, blood dyscrasia, CNS disorders
   6. Drug interactions
      a) Emetine: none significant
      b) Furazolidone: increased pressor effect caused by inhibition of MAO (monoamine oxidase) metabolism when combined with amphetamines, MAO inhibitors, levodopa, tyramine, ephedrine
      c) Iodoquinol: increased binding of iodine to protein, interfering with thyroid function tests, when combined with iodine-containing preparations
      d) Metronidazole
         (1) Warfarin-type anticoagulants: enhanced hypoprothrombinemia
         (2) Disulfiram: acute psychotic reaction and confusion
         (3) Alcohol: flushing, sweating, headache, nausea, vomiting, and abdominal cramps
         (4) Phenobarbital: increased metronidazole metabolism
      e) Pentamidine: increased nephrotoxic effects with aminoglycosides, cisplatin, and amphotericin B
      f) Quinacrine: increased toxicity of primaquine; acute psychotic reaction and confusion when taken with alcohol

C. Nursing diagnoses
   1. Altered protection related to adverse hematologic effects
   2. Altered health maintenance related to cinchonism (quinine)

      3. High risk for fluid volume deficit related to adverse GI effects (antiamebiasis agent)

  D. Nursing implementation factors

      1. Administration procedures

          a) Reduce GI upset by administering chloroquine, primaquine, and quinine with food.

          b) Take seizure precautions when administering chloroquine, hydroxy-chloroquine, mefloquine, or pyrimethamine to susceptible clients.

          c) Refrain from IV administration of emetine.

      2. Daily monitoring and measurements

          a) Assess client's hydration if adverse GI effects occur.

          b) Observe client for signs and symptoms of cinchonism during quinine treatment.

      3. Points for client teaching

          a) Advise client to abstain from strenuous exercise during emetine treatment and for several weeks thereafter.

          b) Explain to client that iodoquinol treatment will falsify results of thyroid function tests for up to 6 months.

          c) Instruct client with amebiasis to avoid reinfection by practicing proper hygiene.

  E. Nursing evaluations

      1. Client's signs and symptoms have decreased.

      2. Client is adequately hydrated.

      3. Client has no symptoms of cinchonism.

      4. Client experiences no adverse CNS effects.

V. Anthelmintic agents

See text pages
_____

  A. Examples: mebendazole (Vermox), thiabendazole (Mintezol), niclosamide (Niclocide), praziquantel (Biltricide), piperazine (Antepar)

  B. Use/mechanism of action: treat infections caused by nematodes, cestodes, or trematodes by acting on parasite microtubules, paralyzing parasite, or interfering with conversion of food to energy

  C. Adverse effects

      1. Most anthelmintic agents: GI upset; some CNS effects, such as headache and dizziness

      2. Mebendazole: fever, leukopenia, hypospermia

      3. Praziquantel: malaise, drowsiness, fatigue, transiently increased AST and ALT levels, macular rash with pruritus

      4. Thiabendazole: tinnitus, hyperirritability, fever, chills, rash, pruritus, urinary odor

D. Contraindications: pregnancy, lactation

E. Precautions: Crohn's disease, ulcerative colitis, hepatic impairment, early childhood, malnutrition, dehydration, anemia

F. Drug interactions: increased metabolism of mebendazole, decreasing its efficacy, when administered with carbamazepine or phenytoin

G. Nursing diagnoses
   1. Pain related to parasitic infection
   2. Potential for injury related to adverse GI effects
   3. Risk for impaired skin integrity related to rash

H. Nursing implementation factors
   1. Administration procedures
      a) Treat all family members for nematode infection to prevent recurrence.
      b) Administer praziquantel with meals to reduce adverse GI effects; explain to client that tablet is bitter and must be swallowed rapidly to avoid gagging or retching.
   2. Daily monitoring and measurements
      a) Monitor hydration if client experiences GI distress.
      b) Obtain prescription for antiemetic or antidiarrheal medications, if needed.
   3. Points for client teaching
      a) Tell client that mebendazole, niclosamide, and thiabendazole tablets should be chewed.
      b) Instruct client to change and wash underclothing and bedding daily until nematodes have been eliminated.
      c) Advise client to wash hands and underneath fingernails after each bowel movement.

I. Nursing evaluations
   1. Client's infection has resolved.
   2. Client's signs and symptoms have disappeared.
   3. Client's skin remains intact.
   4. Client has no adverse GI effects.
   5. Client has no significant adverse CNS effects beyond mild headache successfully managed with analgesic.

VI. Antitubercular agents

See text pages

A. Examples: ethambutol (Myambutol); isoniazid (INH, Nydrazid); rifampin (Rifadin)

B. Use/mechanism of action
   1. Ethambutol: treat tuberculosis and other mycobacterial infections by acting against replicating organisms
   2. Isoniazid: treat tuberculosis and other mycobacterial infections, apparently by inhibiting components of cell wall
   3. Rifampin: treat tuberculosis and other mycobacterial infections by inhibiting RNA synthesis

C. Adverse effects: GI effects (most common); hypersensitivity reactions; optic neuritis (ethambutol), peripheral neuritis (isoniazid at high doses)

D. Contraindications: lactation; optic neuritis and childhood (ethambutol); clinically active hepatitis (rifampin)

E. Precautions: pregnancy, alcoholism, liver or renal impairment

F. Drug interactions
   1. Isoniazid, cycloserine, and ethionamide in combination: additive CNS effects
   2. Aluminum antacids and isoniazid: decreased isoniazid absorption
   3. Rifampin with oral contraceptives, ketoconazole, quinidine, cyclosporine, chloramphenicol, corticosteroids, methadone, oral hypoglycemic agents, warfarin, cardiac glycosides, dapsone: increased metabolism of these agents by rifampin, resulting in reduced efficacy

G. Nursing diagnoses
   1. Anxiety related to diagnosis
   2. Altered respiration related to lung infection
   3. Sensory-perceptual alterations: visual related to optic neuritis
   4. Lack of knowledge related to prevention and treatment of tuberculosis

H. Nursing implementation factors
   1. Administration procedures
      a) Administer rifampin between meals.
      b) Separate administration of isoniazid and an aluminum antacid by at least 1 hour.
   2. Daily monitoring and measurements
      a) Monitor client receiving isoniazid or high-dose ethambutol for signs and symptoms of optic neuritis.
      b) Question client receiving isoniazid about muscle twitching or paresthesia of hands and feet.
   3. Points for client teaching
      a) Tell client receiving isoniazid or ethambutol to report changes in vision.
      b) Caution client that rifampin may discolor urine, sweat, tears, sputum, and feces and that these secretions may stain clothing and soft contact lenses.

I. Nursing evaluations
   1. Client's tuberculosis is in remission.
   2. Client's signs and symptoms have resolved.
   3. Client's vision remains normal.
   4. Client understands and takes preventive measures.

1. The physician has ordered ceftriaxone (Rocephin) for 7-year-old Melissa. Before administering the drug, the nurse should check for:

   a. Abnormal white blood cell count (WBC).
   b. Elevated liver enzymes.
   c. History of penicillin allergy.
   d. History of neuromuscular disease.

2. Mr. Baxter is receiving netilmicin sulfate (Netromycin) to treat peritonitis after emergency repair of a lacerated colon. During the first 48 hours after surgery, it is especially important that the nurse monitor for which evidence of adverse effects?

   a. Slow, shallow respirations
   b. Sudden, extreme temperature elevation
   c. Polyuria and dehydration
   d. Jaundice

3. A client who will be taking tetracycline should be warned to avoid using which of the following within 1 hour of taking the tetracycline?

   a. Cough suppressants
   b. Antacids
   c. Acidic fruit juices
   d. Antihistamines

4. The adult client receiving chloramphenicol (Chloromycetin) for a systemic *Salmonella* infection should be instructed to report which of the following to the physician immediately?

   a. Sore throat and fever
   b. Very low urinary output
   c. Yellow skin color
   d. Ringing in the ears

5. Mr. Everett has been taking erythromycin estolate (Ilosone) for 4 weeks to treat a persistent mycoplasma pneumonia. Which of the following laboratory studies must be monitored regularly for Mr. Everett?

   a. Blood urea nitrogen (BUN) and creatinine
   b. WBC
   c. Liver function
   d. Blood glucose

6. After 1 week of therapy with clindamycin (Cleocin), Mrs. Dolan reports persistent fever of 100°–101°F and severe, foul-smelling diarrhea that includes a great deal of mucus. The nurse should:

   a. Instruct her to avoid dairy products and force fluids.
   b. Suggest use of a kaolin/pectin anti-diarrheal such as Kaopectate.
   c. Suggest use of a systemic antidiarrheal such as loperamide.
   d. Tell her to stop taking clindamycin immediately.

7. A client receiving IV vancomycin (Vancocin) must be monitored frequently for:

   a. Jaundice.
   b. Hearing loss.
   c. Red-green color blindness.
   d. High blood pressure.

8. Betty Franklin has genital herpes, for which oral acyclovir (Zovirax) has been prescribed. It is appropriate to tell her which of the following?

   a. Acyclovir will eliminate the virus and cure her herpes.
   b. Acyclovir prevents recurrence of lesions but does not cure herpes.
   c. Acyclovir speeds healing of lesions but does not prevent future outbreaks.
   d. While taking acyclovir, she is not infectious to others.

9. After being exposed to an influenza A epidemic, Mrs. Grady is given amantadine (Symmetrel) as a preventive measure. She should be told to:

   a. Take the ordered amount as a single daily dose.
   b. Take the drug 1 hour before or 2 hours after a meal.
   c. Take the drug immediately after eating breakfast and dinner.
   d. Take 1 dose at bedtime.

10. Mrs. Harding, who takes glyburide (Micronase) for diabetes mellitus, develops a urinary tract infection with *Candida*. Fluconazole (Diflucan) is prescribed. She must be taught to:

    a. Have orange juice or glucose solution available at all times.

    b. Watch for symptoms of hyperglycemia.

    c. Immediately report any symptoms of secondary bacterial infection.

    d. Report bleeding gums or hematuria immediately.

11. Intravenous pentamidine (Pentam) is used to treat *Pneumocystis carinii* pneumonia in Mr. Griggs, who has AIDS. The nurse should:

    a. Limit Mr. Griggs's fluid intake prior to the infusion.

    b. Keep Mr. Griggs in a supine position during the infusion.

    c. Avoid serving Mr. Griggs dairy products during the therapy.

    d. Administer diphenhydramine before beginning the infusion.

12. The Minter family is being treated with mebendazole (Vermox) for pinworm infestation. They should be told to:

    a. Take the tablets on an empty stomach.

    b. Drink a full glass of milk with each tablet.

    c. Eat more dark green leafy vegetables.

    d. Chew the tablets thoroughly before swallowing them.

ANSWERS

1. Correct answer is c. Up to 10% of clients who are allergic to penicillin have cross-sensitivity to cephalosporins. Clients with a history of penicillin sensitivity must be carefully monitored for allergic reactions to cephalosporins.

    a. Clients with infections often have elevated WBC. Cephalosporins do not commonly cause alterations in WBC.

    b. Elevated liver enzymes indicate liver disease. Cephalosporins are seldom hepatotoxic, so this is not relevant.

    d. Cephalosporins are not known to have adverse neuromuscular effects. Neuromuscular blockade is associated with aminoglycosides.

2. Correct answer is a. Neuromuscular blockade may occur with aminoglycosides. This is a particular concern when they are used after a surgical procedure in which other neuromuscular blocking agents have been used.

    b. Sudden, extreme temperature elevation describes malignant hyperthermia, an anesthesia reaction that occurs during surgery. It is not an adverse effect of aminoglycosides.

    c. Aminoglycosides do not produce increased urinary output. The renal damage caused by aminoglycosides produces increased serum creatinine levels, protein or casts in the urine, and oliguria or anuria.

    d. Aminoglycosides are not likely to be hepatotoxic, so jaundice would not be anticipated.

3. Correct answer is b. Calcium, magnesium, aluminum, and iron form complexes with tetracycline that prevent absorption of the drug.

    a. Cough suppressants often contain alcohol, which is a concern with cephalosporins, not tetracyclines.

    c. Acid pH is not known to alter tetracycline absorption.

    d. No interaction between tetracyclines and antihistamines has been reported.

4. Correct answer is a. Bone marrow suppression is the most common toxic effect of chloramphenicol. When the WBC drops, normal flora in the throat produce infection, resulting in sore throat and fever.

    b. Very low urinary output applies to nephrotoxicity, a common toxicity of cephalosporins and aminoglycosides, not chloramphenicol.

    c. Yellow skin color applies to hepatotoxicity, which is occasionally seen with some penicillins but is not likely with chloramphenicol.

d. Ringing in the ears describes tinnitus, a symptom of ototoxicity, which is a concern with aminoglycosides, not chloramphenicol.

5. Correct answer is c. Cholestatic hepatitis is a rare but serious complication of prolonged erythromycin therapy.

a. BUN and creatinine detect nephrotoxicity, not an anticipated adverse effect of erythromycin. It would be appropriate for the client receiving cephalosporins or aminoglycosides.
b. WBC detects bone marrow suppression, a concern with chloramphenicol, not erythromycin.
d. Erythromycins are not known to alter blood glucose levels.

6. Correct answer is d. These may be symptoms of pseudomembranous colitis, a potentially fatal overgrowth of toxin-producing *Clostridium difficile* organisms. The drug must be discontinued and the physician notified immediately.

a. Avoiding dairy products and forcing fluids is appropriate treatment of antibiotic-induced diarrhea, which is common with clindamycin. However, the presence of foul odor, large amounts of mucus, and fever with the diarrhea suggest the more serious pseudomembranous colitis and must be investigated.
b and **c.** If Mrs. Dolan has pseudomembranous colitis, the use of antidiarrheal drugs is inappropriate. They may mask symptoms while permitting the *C. difficile* infection to worsen.

7. Correct answer is b. Vancomycin is known to be ototoxic, so the client must be monitored for hearing loss. The drug should be discontinued if hearing loss occurs.

a. Jaundice is a sign of hepatotoxicity, which may occur with some penicillins but is not common with vancomycin.
c. Red-green color blindness is seen with optic neuritis caused by ethambutol. It is not an adverse effect of vancomycin.

d. Hypotension is the most likely adverse effect of IV vancomycin. It occurs more frequently when infusion rates are rapid.

8. Correct answer is c. Acyclovir speeds healing and shortens the duration of an outbreak but is not a cure.

a. No drug can eliminate a viral infection. Acyclovir is not a cure.
b. Acyclovir has no effect on the frequency of recurrence of outbreaks. It can only limit the symptoms when an outbreak occurs.
d. As long as lesions are present, Betty can infect others. Acyclovir has no effect on infection transmissibility.

9. Correct answer is c. Amantadine is best absorbed when taken immediately after a meal.

a. Taking a single daily dose would increase the risk of adverse neurologic reactions.
b. Amantadine is one of the few drugs whose absorption is improved by taking it with food.
d. Amantadine may cause insomnia. To avoid this, the last daily dose should be taken a few hours before bedtime.

10. Correct answer is a. Fluconazole interacts with glyburide to increase the risk of hypoglycemia. Mrs. Harding needs to be prepared to treat hypoglycemic reactions with orange juice or other high-glucose products.

b. Hyperglycemia is not anticipated either from fluconazole alone or from the interaction of fluconazole and glyburide.
c. Secondary fungal infections are common when bacterial infections are treated with antibiotics. This occurs because antibiotics decrease the numbers of normal flora that normally inhibit fungal growth. Reducing fungal growth would not increase the risk of bacterial overgrowth.
d. Reporting bleeding gums or hematuria would be necessary only if Mrs. Harding is taking warfarin. Prolonged prothrombin time results from the interaction of warfarin and fluconazole. It does not occur with fluconazole and glyburide.

11. **Correct answer is b.** Severe hypotension or arrhythmias are possible during IV infusion of pentamidine. Maintaining a supine position during infusion will minimize this effect.

   a. Fluids should be forced during pentamidine therapy to decrease the risk of nephrotoxicity.

   c. Hypocalcemia is a potential effect of pentamidine. Limiting intake of dairy products, a major source of calcium, would increase the risk.

   d. Diphenhydramine is often given prior to administering amphotericin B to prevent severe chills. It is not indicated with pentamidine.

12. **Correct answer is d.** Mebendazole tablets should be chewed to enhance the drug's effectiveness.

   a. Food does not interact negatively with mebendazole. It may be taken before or after meals.

   b. There is no particular reason to give milk with mebendazole, although it would not be contraindicated.

   c. Dark green leafy vegetables are high in vitamin K, which should be increased when a drug alters normal GI flora. This is not the case with mebendazole.

10

Antineoplastics and Drugs Affecting the Immune Response

NURSING HIGHLIGHTS

1. The nurse can play a vital role in allaying fears and helping clients to deal with the emotional ups and downs often experienced during chemotherapy.
2. The nurse should remember that teaching may be ineffective at times of great anxiety and stress; under those conditions, client instruction should be limited to essentials, which can be written down for future reference.
3. Body image disturbances caused by alopecia and local tissue damage can cause great distress; the nurse should reassure client that these effects are temporary and can be minimized cosmetically.
4. Nurses can play an important role in health maintenance by educating patients about the importance and timing of immunizations.

GLOSSARY

active immunity—protection against disease that occurs as a result of prior exposure to an infectious agent or its antigens; also called acquired immunity

alkylating agent—a drug that replaces a hydrogen atom with an alkyl group; some antineoplastic agents act upon nucleic acids, disrupting their normal functions

cell cycle, G-phase—the first (G_1) stage of the cell cycle, during which the cell manufactures the enzymes needed for DNA synthesis and the G_2 stage, during which specialized DNA proteins and RNA are synthesized for mitosis

cell cycle, M-phase—the final (mitosis) stage of the cell cycle, during which the cell divides by a process of prophase (clumping of chromosomes), metaphase (lining up of chromosomes at middle of cell), anaphase (separation of chromosomes), and telophase (actual division of cell)

cell cycle, S-phase—the second (synthesis) stage of the cell cycle, during which DNA replication occurs in preparation for mitosis

nadir—the lowest point on a scale, often referring to the time when the blood counts are the lowest

toxoid—a modified or inactivated exotoxin that has lost its toxicity but still has the ability to combine with an antitoxin or stimulate its production

vaccine—a suspension of attenuated or killed bacteria, viruses, or rickettsiae used to prevent, ameliorate, or treat an infectious disease

vesicant—an agent that produces blisters

ENHANCED OUTLINE

I. Antineoplastics

See text pages

A. Alkylating agents
  1. Examples
    a) Nitrogen mustards: chlorambucil (Leukeran), cyclophosphamide (Cytoxan), mechlorethamine (Mustargen), melphalan (Alkeran), uracil mustard
    b) Nitrosoureas: carmustine (BCNU), lomustine (CCNU), streptozocin (Zanosar)
    c) Alkylatorlike agents: busulfan (Myleran), cisplatin (Platinol), pipobroman (Vercyte)
  2. Use/mechanism of action: treat leukemias; non-Hodgkin's lymphomas; multiple myeloma; melanoma; sarcoma; cancer of breast, ovaries, uterus, lung, brain, testes, bladder, prostate, and stomach by disrupting DNA (cell cycle–nonspecific [CCNS])
  3. Adverse effects: bone marrow suppression, consisting of leukopenia (infection), thrombocytopenia (bleeding), and anemia (fatigue); nausea, vomiting, epithelial tissue damage, alopecia

4. Contraindications: pregnancy, lactation, known hypersensitivity; renal or hearing impairment, myelosuppression
5. Precautions: leukopenia, thrombocytopenia, bone marrow tumor
6. Drug interactions
   a) Cyclophosphamide with succinylcholine: prolonged neuromuscular blockade with succinylcholine
   b) Cyclophosphamide with chloramphenicol: reduced conversion of chloramphenicol to active metabolites

B. Antimetabolite agents
1. Examples: cytarabine (Cytosar-U), fluoracil (5-FU), floxuridine (FUDR), mercaptopurine (Purinethol), methotrexate (Mexate), thioguanine
2. Use/mechanism of action: treat acute leukemia; breast cancer; adenocarcinoma of gastrointestinal (GI) tract; non-Hodgkin's lymphomas; squamous cell carcinoma of head, neck, and cervix by disrupting the S-phase of the cell cycle (cell cycle–specific [CCS]), when DNA is synthesized
3. Adverse effects: bone marrow suppression, severe stomatitis, fatigue, hepatotoxicity that may lead to cirrhosis or acute liver atrophy, pneumonitis, pulmonary fibrosis, nephrotoxicity, photosensitivity
4. Contraindications: pregnancy, lactation, known hypersensitivity; blood dyscrasias (methotrexate)
5. Precautions: hepatic impairment, infection, peptic ulcer, ulcerative colitis, extremes of age (methotrexate)
6. Drug interactions
   a) Methotrexate with probenecid, penicillins, salicylates, nonsteroidal anti-inflammatory drugs (NSAIDs): inhibition of methotrexate excretion, increasing risk of toxicity
   b) Methotrexate with cholestyramine: reduced GI absorption of methotrexate
   c) Methotrexate with alcohol: increased methotrexate hepatotoxicity
   d) Methotrexate with live vaccines: increased risk of infection by organism in vaccine
   e) Methotrexate with co-trimoxazole: megaloblastic pancytopenia
   f) Mercaptopurine with allopurinol: increased bone marrow suppression

C. Antibiotic antitumor agents
1. Examples: bleomycin (Blenoxane), dactinomycin (Cosmegen), daunorubicin (Cerubidine), doxorubicin (Adriamycin), mitomycin (Mutamycin), mitoxantrone (Novantrone), plicamycin (Mithramycin)
2. Use/mechanism of action: treat Hodgkin's and non-Hodgkin's lymphomas; testicular cancer; squamous cell carcinoma of head, neck, and cervix; Wilms' tumor; osteogenic sarcoma; rhabdomyosarcoma; soft-tissue sarcoma; breast, ovarian, bladder, and bronchogenic carcinomas; acute leukemias; melanoma; and GI tract carcinomas by disrupting DNA (cell cycle–nonspecific), disrupting S-phase activity (doxorubicin), or disrupting G-phase and S-phase activity (mitomycin)
3. Adverse effects: cardiac toxicity, bone marrow suppression, stomatitis, alopecia, nausea, vomiting, severe tissue damage if extravasated; fever and chills (bleomycin)

      4. Contraindications: pregnancy, myelosuppression, known hypersensitivity

      5. Precautions: serious renal or hepatic impairment, cardiovascular disease, mediastinal radiation therapy

      6. Drug interactions: none significant

D. Plant alkaloids/mitotic inhibitors

      1. Examples: vinblastine (Velban), vincristine (Oncovin), etoposide (VePesid)

      2. Use/mechanism of action: treat Hodgkin's disease, non-Hodgkin's lymphoma, testicular cancer, lymphosarcoma, breast cancer, acute lymphocytic leukemia, Wilms' tumor, and neuroblastoma by disrupting the M-phase or disrupting G_2 phase activity of the cell cycle (CCS) (etoposide)

      3. Adverse effects: neuromuscular abnormalities and peripheral neuropathies, bone marrow suppression, alopecia, severe tissue damage if extravasated (vesicant)

      4. Contraindications: pregnancy, lactation, granulocytopenia from unrelated disease processes, bacterial infection

      5. Precautions: acute uric acid nephropathy, neuromuscular disease

      6. Drug interactions: none significant

E. Hormonal agents

      1. Examples

         a) Estrogens: chlorotrianisene, conjugated estrogens, diethylstilbestrol (DES), ethinyl estradiol

         b) Antiestrogens: tamoxifen (Nolvadex)

         c) Androgens: fluoxymesterone (Halotestin), testolactone (Teslac), testosterone

         d) Antiandrogens: flutamide

         e) Adrenocortical suppressants: aminoglutethimide

         f) Progestins: hydroxyprogesterone (Delalutin); medroxyprogesterone (Provera, Depo-Provera); megestrol (Megace)

         g) Corticosteroids: dexamethasone, hydrocortisone, methylprednisolone, prednisolone, prednisone

         h) Gonadotropin-releasing hormone analogues: leuprolide (Lupron)

      2. Use/mechanism of action: treat prostatic, breast, and endometrial cancers (estrogens and androgens) and lymphocytic leukemias and lymphomas (corticosteroids), probably by interfering with growth-stimulating receptor proteins in hormone-sensitive tumors, thus changing the hormonal environment into one that is unfavorable to cancer cell growth

      3. Adverse effects: same as sections VI,A,3; VI,B,3; and VI,C,3 of Chapter 8

      4. Contraindications: pregnancy, undiagnosed genital bleeding, thrombophlebitis

5. Precautions: epilepsy; migraine; cardiac, renal, or hepatic impairment
6. Drug interactions
   a) Aminoglutethimide with dexamethasone: increased dexamethasone metabolism
   b) Aminoglutethimide with warfarin: increased warfarin metabolism

F. Miscellaneous antineoplastics
   1. Examples: asparaginase (Elspar), dacarbazine (DTIC-Dome), hydroxyurea (Hydrea), interferon alfa-2a (Roferon-A), interferon alfa-2b (Intron A), mitotane (Lysodren), procarbazine (Matulane); investigational drugs and biologic response modifiers
   2. Use/mechanism of action
      a) L-asparaginase: treats acute lymphocytic leukemia by reducing asparagine supplies to tumors that depend on it
      b) Mitotane: treats adrenal cortex carcinoma by an unknown mechanism of action
      c) Procarbazine: treats Hodgkin's disease, perhaps by disrupting S-phase activity
      d) Hydroxyurea: treats melanoma, leukemias, and metastatic ovarian cancer by inhibiting DNA synthesis
      e) Interferons: treat hairy-cell leukemia and AIDS-related Kaposi's sarcoma by exerting antiviral, antiproliferative, and immunomodulatory effects
   3. Adverse effects: central nervous system (CNS) toxicity (procarbazine), flulike syndrome (alpha-interferons), leukopenia (hydroxyurea)
   4. Contraindications: pregnancy, lactation, bacterial infection, pancreatitis, inadequate bone marrow reserve, severe anemia
   5. Precautions: recurrent cardiac arrhythmia, recent myocardial infarction, neuromuscular disease, impaired renal or hepatic function
   6. Drug interactions: none significant

G. Nursing diagnoses
   1. Altered nutrition, less than body requirements, related to adverse GI effects
   2. Altered oral mucous membrane related to stomatitis
   3. Body image disturbance related to alopecia
   4. Potential for infection related to immunosuppression
   5. Fluid volume deficit related to GI effects
   6. Potential for injury related to vesicant properties of antineoplastic drug
   7. Fear related to diagnosis and prognosis
   8. Fatigue related to anemia and anorexia
   9. Diarrhea related to adverse GI effects

H. Nursing implementation factors
   1. Administration procedures
      a) Before giving an antineoplastic, check protocols and physician's orders and be sure that all necessary laboratory results have been received and are within acceptable parameters.
      b) Rotate intravenous (IV) sites and inspect client frequently for tissue damage due to extravasation; client may need port or central line.

  c) Stop infusion of vesicants immediately if extravasation occurs (see Nurse Alert, "Local Tissue Damage Caused by Antineoplastic Agents").

 2. Daily monitoring and measurements

  a) Check client's oral membranes frequently for stomatitis.

  b) Watch client with leukopenia for signs of infection, such as fever, chills, sore throat, malaise, and productive cough.

  c) Avoid intramuscular (IM) injections and venipunctures if thrombocytopenia occurs; watch client for signs of bleeding.

  d) Monitor complete blood cell count (CBC) for abnormalities that suggest development of thrombocytopenia or leukopenia.

 3. Points for client teaching

  a) Tell client to notify physician or nurse if fever, sore throat, unusual bleeding or bruising, or signs of anemia (unusual fatigue or difficulty in breathing) occur.

  b) Teach client appropriate infection control measures, bleeding precautions, and energy-conservation methods.

  c) Advise client to report any of the following signs of jaundice to the physician immediately: yellowing of skin or sclera, right upper quadrant pain, darkened urine, clay-colored stools.

  d) Educate client about the difference between medically established and fringe therapies for cancer.

!   NURSE *ALERT*   !

Local Tissue Damage Caused by Antineoplastic Agents

To protect yourself and the client, you should know which antineoplastic agents can produce blisters and tissue damage if extravasated (the vesicant agents), which may produce hypersensitivity reactions (the irritant agents), and which are relatively innocuous (the nonvesicant agents). Members of these groups are given in the following lists.

Vesicants:	Irritants:	Nonvesicants:
• dacarbazine	• carmustine	• asparaginase
• dactinomycin	• etoposide	• bleomycin
• daunorubicin	• streptozocin	• carboplatin
• doxorubicin		• cisplatin
• mitomycin		• cyclophosphamide
• mitoxantrone		• cytarabine
• nitrogen mustards		• floxuridine
• plicamycin		• fluorouracil
• vinblastine		• ifosfamide
• vincristine		
• vindesine		

e) Answer client's questions, being honest and hopeful.

f) Advise client to buy wig before start of chemotherapy if hair loss is expected.

g) Encourage client who is receiving an antimetabolite to drink abundant fluids.

I. Nursing evaluations
1. X-ray and physical examination reveal tumor or disease regression.
2. Client maintains body weight within acceptable range.
3. Client's mucous membranes are normal.
4. Client has adjusted to hair loss.
5. Client's IV sites show minimal tissue irritation.
6. Client's vomiting is controlled or eliminated.
7. Client is watchful for early signs and symptoms of infection.
8. Client maintains an attitude of realistic hope.
9. Client schedules activities to conserve strength.
10. Client's diarrhea is controlled or eliminated.

II. Immunosuppressants and immunomodulators

See text pages
_____

A. Immunosuppressants
1. Examples: azathioprine (Imuran), cyclosporine (Sandimmune), muromonab-CD3 (Orthoclone OKT3)
2. Use/mechanism of action: prevent rejection after organ transplantation by reducing the immune response through interference with the ability of lymphocytes to produce antibodies and killer T cells, which attack and destroy foreign cells
3. Adverse effects: anorexia, nausea, vomiting, leukopenia, infection, megaloblastic anemia
4. Contraindications: fluid overload, known hypersensitivity
5. Precautions: previous exposure to muromonab-CD3, systemic reaction to an antithymocyte globulin (ATG) skin test
6. Drug interactions
   a) Vaccines, live virus: increased replication of vaccine virus, increased adverse effects, decreased antibody response
   b) Azathioprine with allopurinol: increased azathioprine levels, heightening risk of toxicity
   c) Cyclosporine with androgens, cimetidine, danazol, diltiazem, estrogens, erythromycin, ketoconazole, miconazole: increased cyclosporine levels, heightening risk of toxicity
   d) Cyclosporine with potassium-sparing diuretics, potassium supplements, salt substitutes: increased risk of hyperkalemia
   e) Other immunosuppressants: increased risk of infection and lymphoma

B. Immunomodulators
1. Examples
   a) Marketed agents: interferon alpha-2a (Roferon-A), interferon alpha-2b (Intron A)

      b) Investigational agents: ampligen (Poly IC12U), diethyl dithio carbamate (Imuthiol), Imreg-1, Imreg-2, beta interferon (Betaseron), thymostimuline (TP-1)

  2. Use/mechanism of action: inhibit cell growth and regulate natural killer cells of the immune system by incompletely understood mechanisms

  3. Adverse effects: pruritus, swelling and pain at administration site, flulike symptoms

  4. Contraindications: lactation

  5. Precautions: pregnancy, recent myocardial infarction, arrhythmic disorder

  6. Drug interactions

    a) Vaccines: increased adverse effects of vaccines and decreased antibody response

    b) Radiation therapy or myelosuppressive agent: increased bone marrow suppression

    c) CNS depressants: enhanced CNS effects

    d) Methylxanthines: increased half-life of methylxanthines

C. Nursing diagnoses

  1. Anxiety and fear related to severity of underlying disorder and side effects associated with treatment

  2. Altered nutrition, less than body requirements, related to adverse GI effects

  3. Potential for infection related to immunosuppression

  4. Altered oral mucous membranes related to stomatitis

  5. Impaired skin integrity related to local irritation at administration site

  6. Altered comfort related to pruritus

D. Nursing implementation factors

  1. Administration procedures

    a) Take extraordinary care to maintain aseptic conditions.

    b) Administer adequate fluids to minimize dehydration and lessen risk of urinary tract infection.

  2. Daily monitoring and measurements

    a) Monitor client's vital signs and weight.

    b) Measure client's fluid intake and output.

    c) Monitor client for signs of infection.

    d) Monitor daily blood work.

  3. Points for client teaching

    a) Advise immunosuppressed client to practice excellent hygiene, including dental and mouth care.

    b) Tell client to report immediately any symptoms of infection, including sore throat, malaise, headache, fever, and dysuria.

    c) Caution client to avoid breaking the skin or sustaining other types of trauma.

E. Nursing evaluations
    1. Rejection of transplanted organ is prevented.
    2. Client shows no signs or symptoms of infection.
    3. Client experiences only mild effects of immunosuppression and maintains normal hydration and body weight.
    4. Client is calm and demonstrates adequate knowledge of drug and its effects.
    5. Client maintains intact skin and oral mucous membranes.

III. Vaccines and toxoids

See text pages _____

A. Examples
    1. Vaccines: bacillus Calmette-Guerin (BCG) vaccine, cholera vaccine, typhoid vaccine, pneumococcal vaccine polyvalent (Pneumovax 23), hemophilus B polysaccharide vaccine (Hib-Imune), Hemophilus B with diphtheria toxoid conjugate vaccine (ProHIBiT), hepatitis B vaccine (Recombivax HB), measles (rubeola) virus vaccine, rubella virus vaccine (Meruvax II), mumps virus vaccine (Mumpsvax), poliovirus vaccine, influenza virus vaccine (Fluogen), rabies vaccine
    2. Toxoids: tetanus toxoid, diphtheria toxoid, diphtheria and tetanus toxoid and pertussis vaccine (DTP)

B. Use/mechanism of action: provide active immunity against specific bacterial, viral, or rickettsial disease by stimulating antibody production in response to attenuated organism or toxin

C. Adverse effects: local pain or rash at injection site, mild fever, malaise, nausea, vomiting

D. Contraindications: pregnancy

E. Precautions: immunosuppression, acute infection

F. Drug interactions
    1. Influenza virus with warfarin, theophylline: possible inhibition of warfarin and theophylline clearance
    2. Rabies vaccine with corticosteroids, other immunosuppressants: reduced antibody production

G. Nursing diagnoses
    1. Potential for infection related to causative organism
    2. Pain related to swelling and irritation at injection site

H. Nursing implementation factors
    1. Administration procedures
        a) Most vaccines should be refrigerated and transported with ice packs; only dry ice should be used for transporting polio vaccine.
        b) Most vaccines should be mixed just prior to administration.
        c) Record identification (lot) number of vaccine so that batch can be traced in the event of a severe reaction.
    2. Daily monitoring and measurements: Inspect injection site for local irritation and swelling.

   3. Points for client teaching
      a) Tell client when to return for booster vaccination, if needed.
      b) Advise client for how long the immunization will be effective.
      c) Explain to client that redness and pain at injection site are normal adverse effects.
      d) Caution client to report more severe adverse effects.

I. Nursing evaluations
   1. Titers show that vaccination has been successful.
   2. Client shows only mild tissue irritation at administration site.

1. The client receiving an antimetabolite to treat cancer is at risk for stomatitis. To help prevent this condition, the client should be taught to:
   a. Use a Toothette to clean the teeth after each meal and at bedtime.
   b. Rinse the mouth frequently with hydrogen peroxide solution.
   c. Floss the teeth twice a day.
   d. Use lemon-glycerin swabs to clean the mouth every 2 hours.

2. High-dose methotrexate is used to treat Mr. Foley's lymphoma. To reduce his risk of toxicity, which drug should the nurse anticipate administering?
   a. Aspirin
   b. Leucovorin
   c. Probenecid
   d. Mesna

3. In addition to the usual precautions for a client about to receive antineoplastic therapy, the client who is to receive doxorubicin (Adriamycin) will need baseline studies of:
   a. Hearing.
   b. Pulmonary function.
   c. Cardiac function.
   d. Glucose tolerance.

4. Mrs. Parker will be receiving vincristine (Oncovin) to treat Hodgkin's disease. Which advice should she be given?
   a. Brush her hair vigorously once a day.
   b. Wash her hair daily with baby shampoo.
   c. Anticipate permanent hair thinning or baldness.
   d. Purchase a wig or hairpiece before therapy begins.

5. Mrs. Parker should be monitored for which of the following while she is taking vincristine?
   a. Severe diarrhea
   b. Peripheral neuropathy

   c. Respiratory distress
   d. Masculinizing effects

6. Mrs. Lucas is taking tamoxifen (Nolvadex) for treatment of metastatic breast cancer. She needs to have which of the following more frequently than usual?
   a. Visual acuity testing
   b. Audiometric testing
   c. Dental examinations
   d. Pap smears

7. Mr. Stella is receiving monthly injections of leuprolide (Lupron) to control advanced prostate cancer. He should be warned to anticipate which side effect?
   a. Weight gain
   b. Hot flashes
   c. Frequent urination
   d. Excessive hair growth

8. An appropriate nursing diagnosis to address the adverse effects of interferon alpha-2b (Intron A) is:
   a. Constipation related to GI system response to interferon.
   b. Fluid volume excess related to excessive antidiuretic hormone secretion.
   c. Hypothermia related to toxic effects on the hypothalamus.
   d. Fatigue related to interferon side effects.

9. Mr. Chiang asks the nurse why he must take 5 antineoplastic drugs to treat his leukemia. The best response is:
   a. Because the drugs are very toxic, no one drug can be given in high enough doses to control cancer.
   b. In the late stages of cancer, different drugs must be given because many different types of cells are present.
   c. Each drug acts at a different stage of cell division, so multiple drugs kill more cells.
   d. Several different drugs will be tried until one that is effective for his cancer is identified.

10. An important nursing diagnosis for the client receiving azathioprine (Imuran) to prevent rejection of a transplanted kidney would be:

   a. High risk for infection related to bone marrow depression.
   b. High risk for injury related to central nervous system depression.
   c. Fluid volume excess related to electrolyte imbalances.
   d. Sensory-perceptual alteration: auditory related to ototoxicity.

11. A child should receive the first dose of measles-mumps-rubella vaccine at the age of:

   a. 2 months.
   b. 6 months.
   c. 15 months.
   d. 4 years.

12. Oral polio vaccine, which is a live virus vaccine, should not be administered to:

   a. Infants under 6 months of age.
   b. Anyone who has had a cold within 1 week.
   c. Clients with allergies to seafood.
   d. Children living with immunosuppressed family members.

ANSWERS

1. **Correct answer is a.** Frequent mouth care is helpful for reducing the risk of stomatitis. To avoid damaging fragile mucous membranes, gauze or Toothettes may be used instead of a toothbrush.

   b. Hydrogen peroxide may damage mucous membranes and increase the risk of stomatitis.
   c. During treatment with antineoplastic drugs that suppress bone marrow, flossing should be avoided because it may cause bleeding of the gums and damage mucous membranes.
   d. Glycerin should be avoided because it dries mucous membranes, increasing the risk of cracks or breaks that may not heal while the client is receiving antineoplastics.

2. **Correct answer is b.** Leucovorin, or folinic acid, provides the necessary metabolically active form of folic acid to permit normal cells to survive methotrexate exposure. It must be administered at the correct interval to allow methotrexate to damage rapidly dividing cancer cells but protect normal cells.

   a. Aspirin displaces methotrexate from protein binding sites, elevating serum levels and increasing the risk of toxicity.
   c. Probenecid reduces renal clearance of methotrexate, increasing the risk of toxicity.
   d. Mesna is a uroprotective agent that is used to decrease the risk of hemorrhagic cystitis when certain alkylating agents are given. It is not useful with methotrexate.

3. **Correct answer is c.** Doxorubicin is cardiotoxic. To detect this toxicity, baseline studies of cardiac function are needed for later comparison.

   a. Doxorubicin does not affect hearing. Ototoxicity occurs with aminoglycoside antibiotics.
   b. Pulmonary function studies are appropriate for bleomycin, which is toxic to lungs. They are not essential with doxorubicin.
   d. Doxorubicin is not known to alter glucose tolerance. Some hormonal agents, such as prednisone, do decrease glucose tolerance, producing elevated blood glucose levels.

4. **Correct answer is d.** A wig or hairpiece should be purchased and styled before the hair is lost so it can be matched to the client's hair. This will make the switch to the wig less obvious.

   a and b. Vigorous hair brushing and daily shampooing are often tried by clients who believe that increasing circulation to the scalp will delay or prevent hair loss. Actually, vigorous brushing and frequent washing increase hair loss.
   c. Drug-induced hair loss is seldom permanent. When therapy is completed the hair usually grows back, although it is often a different color or texture.

5. **Correct answer is b.** The vinca alkaloids are neurotoxic. Peripheral neuropathy is a common adverse effect.

a. Diarrhea is common with many antineoplastics, but constipation occurs with vinca alkaloids, as a result of autonomic neuropathy.
c. Respiratory distress is anticipated with bleomycin. It is not a common toxicity of vinca alkaloids.
d. Masculinizing effects result from androgens. They are not expected with vinca alkaloids.

6. **Correct answer is a.** Tamoxifen can cause irreversible decreases in visual acuity. Vision changes may require that the drug be stopped.

b. Ototoxicity is seldom seen with tamoxifen. This is appropriate for loop diuretics or aminoglycoside antibiotics.
c. Tamoxifen does not have adverse effects on teeth or gums. This would be appropriate for phenytoin.
d. Tamoxifen does not increase the risk of cervical or uterine cancers, so there is no reason for more frequent Pap smears.

7. **Correct answer is b.** Hot flashes are the most common side effect of leuprolide, occurring in up to 70% of clients.

a. Some clients experience nausea, vomiting, or anorexia, which may lead to weight loss. Weight gain is not expected.
c. Leuprolide does not cause more frequent urination. It may, in fact, cause some fluid retention and peripheral edema.
d. Leuprolide reduces testosterone levels after the first few days, decreasing the growth of body hair.

8. **Correct answer is d.** A flulike syndrome, with muscle aches, fatigue, and fever, is the most common adverse effect of interferon. Fatigue may be the dose-limiting toxic effect.

a. Diarrhea is a more likely effect of interferon. A nursing diagnosis of constipation would be more appropriate for vinca alkaloids.

b. Fluid volume deficit is a more likely adverse effect, secondary to diarrhea, nausea, and anorexia. Interferon does not cause antidiuretic hormone excess.
c. Fever is more likely with interferon, as part of the flulike syndrome that is a common adverse effect. This nursing diagnosis would be appropriate for clients taking phenothiazines to control nausea.

9. **Correct answer is c.** The actions of different antineoplastic drugs affect cells at different points in cell division. The cancer cells in the body are at various points in the cell cycle. If several drugs with different actions are given, more cancer cells can be destroyed by a single course of chemotherapy.

a. Strategies for managing drug toxicities have been developed, permitting high doses to be used. Dosages are not necessarily reduced when multiple drugs are given.
b. Multidrug regimens are used regardless of whether treatment occurs early or late in the progression of the cancer.
d. Individual cancers do not differ in susceptibility to specific drugs. Cancer cells differ in susceptibility because they are at different points in the cell cycle.

10. **Correct answer is a.** The primary adverse reaction to the immunosuppressant agent azathioprine is bone marrow depression, which causes leukopenia. The decreased white blood cell count increases the client's risk of infection.

b. Central nervous system depression is not an expected effect of azathioprine.
c. Electrolyte imbalances are a common adverse effect of cyclosporine. They are not expected with azathioprine.
d. Ototoxicity is not an expected effect of azathioprine. Retinopathy with visual deficits does sometimes occur.

11. **Correct answer is c.** Maternal antibodies present before the age of 15 months would destroy the vaccine, preventing development of the child's own antibodies. By 15 months of age, maternal antibodies are lost and the child's own immune system produces antibodies to the 3 viruses.

a and b. Vaccine given at 2 or 6 months would be destroyed by maternal antibodies, leaving the child unprotected after the age of 15 months.

d. A second (booster) dose of vaccine after the age of 4 years is recommended.

12. **Correct answer is d.** The client sheds live virus for 3–4 weeks after immunization with live virus vaccine. An immunosuppressed family member may be unable to produce antibodies to this virus and can become infected. Persons who are considered immunosuppressed include those receiving immunosuppressants to prevent rejection of transplanted organs or as chemotherapy for cancer and those infected with the HIV virus.

a. Oral polio vaccine is generally started at the age of 2 months.

b. Vaccines are rarely given during a febrile illness, since it is not possible to distinguish between a reaction to the vaccine and the illness. A cold is not a contraindication as long as there is no fever.

c. Seafood allergies predict iodine allergy. They have no relevance to vaccines, which do not contain iodine.

11

Nutrition and Electrolyte Therapy

NURSING HIGHLIGHTS

1. The nurse should pay considerable attention to educating client and family members about proper diet and basic nutritional requirements.
2. The nurse should be aware that being deprived of the pleasure of food can be a significant cause of depression or mood changes in clients receiving parenteral or enteral feedings.

GLOSSARY

electrolyte—a substance that dissociates in solution into cations and anions and thus can conduct electricity

HHNC (hyperosmolar, hyperglycemic nonketotic coma)—a metabolic complication of prolonged parenteral nutrition caused by trace metal deficiencies

homeostasis—the stability of an organism's normal physiologic state

ENHANCED OUTLINE

I. Enteral and parenteral agents

See text pages
_____

A. Enteral agents
1. Examples (more than 80 available)
   a) Elemental formulations (Flexical, Vital, Vivonex): require minimal digestion and produce minimal residue
   b) Polymeric formulations (Compleat-B, Ensure, Isocal, Magnacal, Osmolite, Portagen, Sustacal): provide complex nutrient support for clients who have functioning gastrointestinal (GI) tracts and do not need a specialized formulation
   c) Modular formulations/single nutrient formulas (protein [Amin-aid, Casec, Hepatic-Aid]; carbohydrate [Controlyte, Polycose]; or fat [MCT Oil]): provide specialized nutrient support; may be added to elemental or polymeric formulation
   d) Altered amino acid formulations: meet special needs of clients with genetic disorders of metabolism or acquired disorders of nitrogen accumulation (cirrhosis or chronic renal failure) and of clients who are catabolic as a result of injury or infection

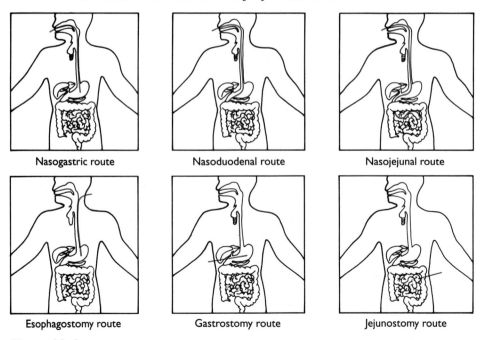

Nasogastric route   Nasoduodenal route   Nasojejunal route

Esophagostomy route   Gastrostomy route   Jejunostomy route

Figure 11–1
Enteral Feeding Routes

2. Use/mechanism of action: treat malnutrition or anorexia by providing necessary nutrients for clients who require nutrient supplementation
3. Adverse effects: diarrhea, cramping, nausea, aspiration pneumonia, constipation; dumping syndrome, caused by too-rapid feeding, consisting of nausea, vomiting, cramping, diarrhea, and malabsorption
4. Contraindications: adynamic ileus, intestinal obstruction, intractable vomiting; esophageal fistulas (with nasogastric tube)
5. Precautions: malabsorption problems
6. Drug interactions: possible gastric obstruction due to interaction of aluminum-based antacids and enteral feeding formulas

B. Parenteral agents
1. Examples (total parenteral nutrition [TPN]): protein-sparing nutrition, peripheral-vein TPN (PTPN), central-vein hyperalimentation
2. Use/mechanism of action: provide complete nutrition to clients whose GI tract is dysfunctional
3. Adverse effects: infection, azotemia, cholelithiasis in children, dehydration from osmotic diuresis, electrolyte imbalance, hyperammonemia, HHNC (hyperosmolar, hyperglycemic nonketotic coma), hyperphosphatemia or hypophosphatemia, hypocalcemia, hypomagnesemia, rebound hypoglycemia, trace element deficiencies (see Nurse Alert, "Trace Element Deficiencies"), essential fatty acid deficiency (see Nurse Alert, "Essential Fatty Acid Deficiency")
4. Contraindications: none
5. Precautions: immunosuppression
6. Drug interactions: none

! NURSE ALERT !

Trace Element Deficiencies

Long-term parenteral feeding increases the risk that a client will develop trace element deficiencies. Be alert to the following signs and symptoms:

Trace Element	Signs and Symptoms
• Chromium	• Neuropathy, confusion, impaired glucose tolerance, ataxia
• Copper	• Decrease in red and white blood cells, hair and skeletal abnormalities, defective tissue growth
• Iodine	• Goiter, cretinism, impaired thyroid functioning
• Manganese	• Defective growth, nausea, vomiting, weight loss, skin rash, ataxia, seizures, and other CNS disturbances
• Molybdenum	• Increased heart rate, tachypnea, headache, nausea, vomiting, edema, malaise, disorientation, coma
• Selenium	• Muscle aches, cardiomyopathy, retarded growth, changes in pigmentation, edema, liver tissue necrosis and fibrosis
• Zinc	• Nausea, vomiting, diarrhea, weakness, anorexia, growth retardation, anemia, hepatosplenomegaly, hypogeusia, rash, depression, defective wound healing, eye lesions

C. Nursing diagnoses
1. Diarrhea related to enteral feeding
2. Anxiety related to intubation procedures
3. Potential for infections related to catheter bacterial seeding
4. Altered role performance related to depression at loss of normal physical and social gratifications of eating

D. Nursing implementation factors
1. Administration procedures
   a) Discard lipid emulsions that have separated.
   b) Change TPN tubing rapidly, with client supine and exhaling against closed glottis.
2. Daily monitoring and measurements
   a) Check client's vital signs and weight.
   b) Measure temperature and report elevations immediately.
   c) Monitor blood urea nitrogen (BUN), complete blood count (CBC), and serum electrolyte levels.
   d) Measure blood and urine glucose.
   e) Measure fluid intake and output in client receiving enteral feeding and check for edema.
3. Points for client teaching
   a) Advise client to alleviate thirst by rinsing mouth, sucking on ice, or using sugarless candy.
   b) Suggest that client who is receiving enteral or parenteral feeding at home maintain normal social interaction by joining family members at mealtimes.
   c) Teach client and family members what to do if solution is aspirated or tube comes out.

E. Nursing evaluations
1. Client's nutritional status is maintained or improved.
2. Client maintains normal hydration.
3. Client shows no signs of infection.
4. Client accepts tube feeding and sucks on ice and sugarless candy to relieve thirst and alleviate desire for food.

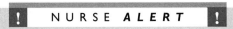

! NURSE *ALERT* !

Essential Fatty Acid Deficiency

Usually, the first sign of this parenteral feeding complication is flaky red skin lesions on the scalp, arms, and legs. Growth retardation may occur in children. Other signs include thrombocytopenia, increased hemolysis, and impaired wound healing.

II. Electrolyte replacement

A. Potassium

    1. Examples: potassium bicarbonate (K-Lyte); potassium chloride (Kaochlor, Slow-K); potassium gluconate (Kaon); potassium phosphate (Neutra-Phos-K)

    2. Use/mechanism of action: restore homeostasis through the use of intracellular fluid electrolytes

    3. Adverse effects: nausea, vomiting, cramps, diarrhea; hyperkalemia, including listlessness, confusion, flaccid paralysis, paresthesia, electrocardiogram (ECG) changes, hypotension leading to peripheral vascular collapse, cardiac arrhythmias, heart block, possible cardiac arrest

    4. Contraindications: renal dysfunction, acute dehydration, hyperkalemia, metabolic acidosis, adrenal insufficiency

    5. Precautions: pregnancy, lactation

    6. Drug interactions: increased risk of hyperkalemia with potassium-sparing diuretics and ACE (angiotensin-converting enzyme) inhibitors

B. Calcium

    1. Examples: calcium carbonate (Os-Cal 500), calcium chloride, calcium citrate (Citracal), calcium glubionate (Neo-Calglucon Syrup), calcium gluconate (Kalcinate), calcium lactate

    2. Use/mechanism of action: restore homeostasis through the use of extracellular fluid electrolytes

    3. Adverse effects: renal calculi; hypercalcemia, including drowsiness, lethargy, muscle weakness, headache, constipation, metallic taste in mouth; severe hypercalcemia, including cardiac arrhythmias, cardiac arrest, coma

    4. Contraindication: hypercalcemia

    5. Precautions: sarcoidosis, renal or cardiac disease, respiratory acidosis, respiratory failure

    6. Drug interactions: cardiac arrhythmias with cardiac glycosides; reduced effectiveness of calcium channel blockers

C. Magnesium

    1. Example: magnesium sulfate

    2. Use/mechanism of action: restore homeostasis through the use of intracellular fluid electrolytes

    3. Adverse effects: hypermagnesemia, including sedation, confusion, muscle weakness, respiratory muscle paralysis, hypotension

    4. Contraindications: hypermagnesemia

    5. Precautions: renal dysfunction

    6. Drug interactions: enhanced neuromuscular blockade with decamethonium, succinylcholine, d-tubocurarine; increased CNS effects with barbiturates, narcotics, hypnotics, systemic anesthetics

D. Sodium

    1. Examples: sodium chloride, sodium bicarbonate injection, sodium lactate injection

    2. Use/mechanism of action: restore homeostasis through the use of extracellular fluid electrolytes

See text pages

3. Adverse effects: hypernatremia, including edema, hypertonicity, red flushed skin, dry sticky mucous membranes, thirst, elevated temperature, decreased urination
4. Contraindications: severe renal and cardiac disease
5. Precautions: renal impairment, congestive heart failure, edema
6. Drug interactions: increased renal clearance of tetracyclines; increased half-lives of quinidine, amphetamines, ephedrine, pseudoephedrine

E. Nursing diagnoses
   1. Potential fluid and electrolyte imbalances
   2. Altered thought processes related to adverse central nervous system (CNS) effects of potassium or calcium

F. Nursing implementation factors
   1. Administration procedures
      a) Administer oral potassium with meals, and tell client not to chew or crush tablets.
      b) Avoid intramuscular (IM) or intravenous (IV) push administration of potassium.
      c) Give electrolytes mixed in IV solutions and change administration site if redness or swelling occurs.
   2. Daily monitoring and measurements
      a) Measure serum electrolytes and fluid intake and output.
      b) Assess client's electrocardiogram (ECG).
   3. Points for client teaching
      a) Discuss with client an appropriate diet that will prevent electrolyte deficiencies.
      b) Reassure client that even if he/she finds wax tablet in stools, potassium has still been absorbed.

G. Nursing evaluations
   1. Client's electrolyte levels are within normal limits.
   2. Client maintains normal hydration.
   3. Client maintains normal bowel pattern.

III. Vitamins and minerals

See text pages
_____

A. Fat-soluble vitamins
   1. Examples: A (beta carotene), D (cholecalciferol [D_3], ergocalciferol [D_2]), E, K (menadiol [synthetic K_3], phytonadione [equivalent to K_1])
   2. Use/mechanism of action
      a) Vitamin A: treat night blindness; treat conditions associated with vitamin A deficiency, including hyperkeratosis, growth retardation, xerophthalmia, keratomalacia, and weakness by stimulating basal epithelial cells to produce mucus-secreting or keratinizing tissues

b) Vitamin D: treat rickets, chronic hypocalcemia and hypophosphatemia, osteodystrophy, and osteomalacia in adults; prevent and treat vitamin D deficiency states and tetany by helping to metabolize calcium and phosphorus

c) Vitamin E: prevent and treat vitamin E deficiency, probably by protecting fatty acids and other oxygen-sensitive substances from oxidation and by decreasing platelet aggregation

d) Vitamin K: promote clotting and treat hypoprothrombinemia by activating clotting precursors

3. Adverse effects

a) Vitamin A: fatigue; malaise; lethargy; abdominal distress; visual disturbances; dry skin, nose, and mouth; inflamed oral mucous membranes; hair loss

b) Vitamin D: calcification of soft tissue, demineralization of bone, nausea, vomiting, anorexia, headache, weakness, diarrhea, constipation

c) Vitamin E (high doses): GI distress, fatigue, weakness, headache, blurred vision, rash

d) Vitamin K: nausea, vomiting, headache when administered by oral route, flushing, dizziness, rapid and weak pulse, hypotension, dyspnea, cyanosis, chest pain when administered by rapid IV; hyperbilirubinemia and jaundice in infants

4. Contraindications: known hypersensitivity

5. Precautions: heart disease, renal calculi, arteriosclerosis, cardiac glycoside therapy (all with ergocalciferol)

6. Drug interactions

a) Vitamin A: decreased absorption with mineral oil

b) Vitamin D: decreased absorption with mineral oil, cholestyramine, cholestipol hydrochloride

c) Vitamin E: reduced anticoagulant effects of warfarin with high doses of vitamin E; reduced hematologic response to iron in treating anemia

d) Vitamin K: antagonism of anticoagulant effects of coumarin

B. Water-soluble vitamins

1. Examples: B-complex (thiamine [B_1], riboflavin [B_2], nicotinic acid or niacin [B_3], pyridoxine [B_6], para-aminobenzoic acid [PABA], pantothenic acid, biotin, choline, inositol, folic acid, cyanocobalamin [B_{12}]), C (ascorbic acid)

2. Use/mechanism of action

a) Thiamine: treat disorders associated with thiamine deficiency, including beriberi, Wernicke's encephalopathy, peripheral neuritis, and pellagra, by combining with adenosine triphosphate to form thiamine pyrophosphate, which acts as a coenzyme in carbohydrate metabolism

b) Riboflavin: treat riboflavin deficiencies, which manifest as digestive disorders, burning in skin and eyes, inflammation and cracking around mouth, inflammation of tongue, scaly dermatitis around nose, headache, and forgetfulness, by assisting in glycogenolysis, tissue respiration, and lipid metabolism; helping to maintain red blood cell (RBC) integrity; and lowering serum cholesterol and triglyceride levels

  c) Nicotinic acid: treat pellagra and help treat hyperlipidemia by carrying hydrogen molecules during tissue respiration, glycogenolysis, and lipid metabolism

  d) Pyridoxine: treat deficiencies occurring with alcoholism, uremia, and malabsorption syndromes and treat deficiencies associated with administration of certain drugs, including isoniazid, cycloserine, hydralazine, ethionamide, penicillamine, and oral contraceptives, by participating in amino acid, carbohydrate, and lipid metabolism and helping to produce several neurotransmitters and proteins

  e) Vitamin C: treat scurvy and acidify urine by helping to form collagen in all fibrous tissue, assisting in carbohydrate metabolism, and probably stimulating connective tissue fibroblasts, promoting tissue repair

 3. Adverse effects

  a) Thiamine: nausea, anxiety, sweating; skin rash, pruritus, or wheezing after large IV dose

  b) Nicotinic acid: rash, pruritus, and wheezing after IV administration; elevated serum levels of glucose and uric acid, liver toxicity, and cardiac arrhythmias at high doses

  c) Pyridoxine: sensory neuropathy with long-term administration of high doses

  d) Ascorbic acid: diarrhea and renal calculi at high doses

 4. Contraindications: hepatic dysfunction, active peptic ulcer disease, severe hypotension

 5. Precautions: gallbladder disease, diabetes, gout, history of renal calculi

 6. Drug interactions

  a) Thiamine: enhanced effect of neuromuscular blocking agents

  b) Riboflavin: impaired absorption with alcohol use; false elevations of urinary catecholamines

  c) Niacin: rhabdomyolysis and myopathy with lovastatin

  d) Pyridoxine: increased levodopa metabolism

  e) Vitamin C: increased iron absorption; decreased warfarin effectiveness

C. Minerals

 1. Examples (trace elements): chromium (Chroma-Pak); copper (Coppertrace); fluoride (Luride, Pediaflor Drops); iodine (SSKI Solution); manganese (Manganese Gluconate); molybdenum (Molypale, Molypen); selenium (Selenitrace); zinc (Orazinc)

 2. Use/mechanism of action

  a) Chromium: prevent chromium deficiency in clients receiving long-term TPN by helping to regulate lipoprotein metabolism and glucose utilization, potentiating action of insulin, and regulating tertiary structures of proteins and nucleic acids

b) Copper: prevent copper deficiency in clients receiving long-term TPN or consuming vegetarian diets; prevent and treat deficiency in clients with disorders that affect copper absorption or excretion, including burns, cancer, nephrosis, and sprue by participating in RBC and white blood cell (WBC) formation, elastin and collagen synthesis, cellular energy production, and glucose and catecholamine metabolism

c) Fluoride: prevent dental caries and desensitize dentin by increasing resistance of teeth to dental caries and acid; increase bone density and relieve bone pain in metabolic and neoplastic bone disease by increasing skeletal mass

d) Iodine: treat goiter and hypothyroidism caused by iodine deficiency, suppress mild forms of hyperthyroidism and thyroid crisis, prepare thyroid clients for thyroidectomy, and induce expectoration by helping to manufacture thyroid hormones T_4 and T_3

e) Manganese: prevent manganese deficiency in clients receiving long-term TPN by helping to activate metalloenzymes and enzymes involved in carbohydrate, protein, and lipid metabolism

f) Molybdenum: prevent molybdenum deficiency in clients receiving long-term TPN by serving as component of aldehyde oxidase, sulfite oxidase, and xanthine oxidase, which participate in many metabolic reactions

g) Selenium: prevent selenium deficiency in clients receiving long-term TPN and in clients with cancer by helping to protect cell membranes and structures from oxidative destruction due to peroxides

h) Zinc: treat zinc deficiency and prevent zinc deficiency in clients receiving long-term TPN by helping to form metalloenzymes and metalloproteins; stabilizing cell membranes; participating in protein and RNA metabolism; interacting with insulin; maintaining arterial wall homeostasis; and assisting in cell growth and proliferation

3. Adverse effects
   a) Chromium: nausea, vomiting, gastric ulceration, rash, joint swelling, bronchospasm, convulsions, coma, kidney and liver damage
   b) Copper: diarrhea, lethargy, altered behavior, diminished reflexes, photophobia, liver and kidney damage
   c) Fluoride: nausea, vomiting, diarrhea, abdominal pain, nervous system hyperirritability, hypocalcemia-related paresthesia and tetany, hypoglycemia, cardiac and respiratory failure, rash, tooth discoloration
   d) Iodine: metallic taste, skin lesions, eyelid swelling, increased salivation, iodide goiter formation, bloody diarrhea, fever, depression; mouth, gum, salivary gland tenderness; hypersensitivity reactions
   e) Manganese: anorexia, diarrhea, headache, parkinsonian symptoms
   f) Molybdenum: goutlike symptoms

g) Selenium: alopecia, skin lesions, GI irritation, depression, garlic odor of breath and sweat; organ failure and death with acute poisoning

h) Zinc: nausea, vomiting, diarrhea, stomach irritation, gastric ulceration, elevated serum amylase levels, hypothermia, hypotension

4. Contraindications: previous allergic reactions

5. Precautions: history of seizures in client receiving high doses of chromium or fluoride, decreased renal or hepatic clearance

6. Drug interactions: impaired absorption of tetracyclines with zinc

D. Nursing diagnoses

1. Potential for injury related to soft-tissue calcification (high-dose vitamin)

2. Altered protection related to vasodilation (nicotinic acid)

3. Impaired tissue integrity related to adverse integumentary effects (vitamin A)

4. Sensory-perceptual alterations: visual related to adverse CNS effects (copper)

E. Nursing implementation factors

1. Administration procedures

a) Refrain from IV administration of vitamin E.

b) Give thiamine and riboflavin with food.

c) Dilute liquid mineral preparations well in advance of administration to decrease GI irritation and improve taste.

d) Do not keep a parenteral solution that contains minerals for more than 24 hours after mixing.

2. Daily monitoring and measurements

a) Monitor client's fat-soluble vitamin intake from food and other sources to avoid toxicity.

b) Assess client's usual patterns of diet and sun exposure to avoid overadministration of vitamin D.

c) Be aware that during vitamin C therapy, client with diabetes may have a false-negative result to a glucose oxidase test or a false-positive result to a glucose level test done with a cupric sulfate tablet.

d) Watch for signs of mineral-induced toxicity, especially in clients with renal or hepatic dysfunction.

e) Monitor client receiving mineral therapy for decreases in blood pressure or changes in body temperature.

3. Points for client teaching

a) Teach client the recommended daily allowance (RDA) and food sources of water-soluble vitamins.

b) Advise client taking fat-soluble vitamins to avoid toxicity by reading labels on containers of prepared foods.

✔ CLIENT TEACHING CHECKLIST ✔

Important Points to Consider about Vitamin Therapy

Clients often believe exaggerated popular claims about the benefits of vitamins, particularly when administered in megadoses. Important teaching points to cover with the client include the following:

✔ Although vitamin deficiencies do cause diseases, self-treatment with megadoses is never an appropriate approach to a medical problem; always consult a physician or a nutritionist.

✔ Vitamins A, D, and B$_6$ can be toxic in excessive doses. Very large doses of vitamin C can cause stones to form in urine.

✔ Since vitamins lose their potency rapidly, check expiration dates and buy small quantities.

✔ Vitamins from "natural sources" are more expensive than synthesized vitamins but are not more therapeutic.

c) Provide client with guidelines on choosing and self-administering vitamins (see Client Teaching Checklist, "Important Points to Consider about Vitamin Therapy").
d) Teach client to deal with side effects of mineral therapy, such as mouth and gum tenderness.
e) Instruct client to prevent GI irritation by taking minerals, except zinc and fluoride, during or immediately after meals.

F. Nursing evaluations
1. Client describes the importance of fruits, vegetables, and whole grain products in preventing mineral deficiencies.
2. Client's diet and vitamin therapy have been coordinated to avoid vitamin overdose.
3. Client experiences only mild flushing with nicotinic acid therapy.

1. Mr. Mason is receiving 240 ml of a poly-meric formulation via nasogastric tube every 6 hours. When his 6:00 A.M. feeding is due, his gastric residual is 150 ml. The nurse should:

   a. Delay the feeding and recheck the resid-ual in 1 hour.
   b. Administer the feeding over 1 hour if bowel sounds are present.
   c. Place Mr. Mason on his left side during the feeding.
   d. Withhold the feeding and notify the physician.

2. While receiving tube feedings, Mr. Mason has persistent diarrhea that standard nurs-ing measures have not relieved. To help identify the cause, the nurse should evalu-ate the results of which laboratory study?

   a. Serum transferrin
   b. Serum albumin
   c. Blood glucose
   d. Urine osmolarity

3. While preparing to administer a parenteral fat emulsion solution, the nurse observes a thin clear layer at the top of the solution. The nurse should:

   a. Agitate the bottle to mix the solution thoroughly.
   b. Warm the solution by setting the bottle in a warm water bath.
   c. Administer the solution through a line with an in-line filter.
   d. Discard the solution.

4. Mr. Roscoe is scheduled to begin receiving total parenteral nutrition (TPN) with a solu-tion of 25% glucose and amino acids. The nurse should anticipate administering which of the following during the first 48 hours of this therapy?

   a. A diuretic
   b. Intramuscular vitamin B_{12}

   c. Regular insulin
   d. Prophylactic antibiotics

5. The client who will be maintained at home on total parenteral nutrition (TPN) should be taught to:

   a. Rinse the mouth every 2 hours with an antimicrobial mouthwash.
   b. Join the family at the table for meal-times.
   c. Avoid the sight and odor of food.
   d. Perform isometric exercises to prevent muscle atrophy.

6. Oral potassium supplements should be administered:

   a. With meals.
   b. On an empty stomach.
   c. At bedtime.
   d. Early in the day.

7. Mrs. Fisher is taking oral calcium supple-ments to treat osteoporosis. She should be told to limit her intake of:

   a. Citrus juices.
   b. Bran.
   c. Red meat.
   d. Dairy products.

8. Mrs. Billings is admitted with eclampsia. She receives IM magnesium sulfate to pre-vent seizures. To detect early signs of hyper-magnesemia, the nurse should frequently check Mrs. Billings's:

   a. Capillary refill time.
   b. Visual acuity.
   c. Pupil responses.
   d. Deep tendon reflexes.

9. A sign of vitamin A deficiency is:

   a. Night blindness.
   b. Inflammation of the tongue.
   c. Petechial rash.
   d. Pathologic fractures.

10. An appropriate nursing diagnosis for the client receiving high doses of vitamin A is:

 a. Diarrhea related to altered intestinal mucosa.

 b. Fluid volume excess related to altered sodium balance.

 c. Impaired swallowing related to enlargement of the thyroid gland.

 d. Impaired skin integrity related to drying effects of vitamin A.

11. Many drug overdoses are treated by acidifying the urine to promote drug excretion. To accomplish this, the nurse may be directed to administer:

 a. Calcium carbonate.

 b. Vitamin K.

 c. Vitamin C.

 d. Sodium bicarbonate.

ANSWERS

1. Correct answer is a. Gastric residuals over 100 ml indicate delayed gastric emptying. Delaying the feeding for 1 hour should allow the stomach to empty. The client should also be assessed for factors that slow gastric emptying.

 b. Administering additional feeding when the stomach is not emptying effectively will further delay gastric emptying. The stomach should be allowed to empty before the next feeding.

 c. Positioning on the left side will further delay gastric emptying. To promote gastric emptying, the client should be on the right side.

 d. This action is premature. The delay in gastric emptying may be a transient problem. If large gastric residuals persist, the physician should be informed.

2. Correct answer is b. Low serum albumin levels are associated with malabsorption, which may cause persistent diarrhea.

 a. Serum transferrin levels are used to evaluate adequacy of dietary protein intake or

ability to utilize iron. Neither is related to the causes of diarrhea.

 c. Changes in blood glucose are not associated with diarrhea.

 d. Urine osmolarity is used to evaluate hydration. Dehydration is more likely to cause constipation than diarrhea.

3. Correct answer is d. If oils have separated out, the solution should not be used.

 a. Lipid emulsion solutions should never be agitated. Agitation could cause fat globules to aggregate.

 b. Lipid emulsions should not be warmed. This method is acceptable for dissolving crystals in mannitol solutions, but it is not used for any other parenteral solution.

 c. In-line filters cannot be used for fat emulsions because the fat particles are too large to pass through the filter.

4. Correct answer is c. When high-glucose solutions are administered, clients often need supplemental insulin during the first few days to prevent hyperglycemia.

 a. The high osmolarity of TPN solutions may lead to dehydration. Diuretics would worsen this effect.

 b. When enteral nutrition is used, clients who lack the intrinsic factor necessary for absorbing B_{12} may need injections of the vitamin. Total parenteral solutions contain the necessary vitamins, including B_{12}.

 d. Strict sterile technique is used to reduce the risk of infection when TPN is used. Antibiotics would be initiated only if there was evidence of infection.

5. Correct answer is b. For many families, mealtime is a primary time for social interaction. To promote normal interaction, the client should join the family at mealtimes and join in conversation.

 a. Antimicrobial mouthwashes are drying to oral mucosa. This would put the client at risk for cracking of lips and mucous membranes and could increase thirst sensation.

c. Although the sight and smell of food may stimulate appetite and cause the client to miss eating, it can also stimulate salivation, which helps reduce dry mouth and thirst. For most clients, the social benefits of being with the family outweigh any feeling of loss related to the inability to eat.
d. Aerobic exercise would be more beneficial in maintaining muscle tone and cardiovascular function. Isometric exercise has no cardiovascular benefits and may involve the Valsalva maneuver, which has adverse cardiovascular effects.

6. **Correct answer is a.** Potassium is very irritating to the mucous membranes that line the GI tract. Food helps prevent this irritation.

   b. Taking potassium on an empty stomach increases the risk of GI irritation.
   c. Medications that cause sedation should be taken at bedtime. This is not a concern with potassium.
   d. Medications that cause diuresis should be taken early in the day to prevent frequent nighttime wakenings. This is not a problem with potassium.

7. **Correct answer is b.** Although bran is useful for preventing constipation, it interferes with calcium absorption.

   a and **c.** Neither citrus juices nor red meats contain substances that interact with calcium.
   d. Dairy products are often fortified with vitamin D, which actually promotes calcium absorption. Clients who need calcium supplements should be encouraged to consume dairy products.

8. **Correct answer is d.** Hypermagnesemia causes muscle weakness and hyporeflexia. Decreased deep-tendon reflexes are an early sign.

   a. Capillary refill time evaluates oxygenation and hydration. Hydration is not

affected by magnesium. Although hypermagnesemia may cause shallow breathing, this does not alter capillary refill until late stages.
b. Visual changes are not associated with magnesium overdose.
c. Pupil changes reflect increased intracranial pressure, which is not associated with magnesium excess.

9. **Correct answer is a.** Vitamin A is important for maintaining the health of the rods and cones in the retina, which are responsible for adaptation to dim light.

   b. Tongue inflammation is a sign of riboflavin (B_2) deficiency.
   c. Petechial rash is a sign of vitamin C deficiency.
   d. Pathologic fractures are a sign of vitamin D deficiency.

10. **Correct answer is d.** Drying of the skin and mucous membranes is the most common adverse effect of large doses of vitamin A.

    a. The diarrhea that occurs with vitamin A deficiency causes changes in the mucous membranes lining the intestine.
    b. Vitamin A does not influence sodium balance.
    c. Enlargement of the thyroid gland occurs with alterations in iodine balance. It is not caused by vitamin A.

11. **Correct answer is c.** Vitamin C, or ascorbic acid, is commonly used to acidify the urine.

    a. Calcium is excreted in the urine but does not alter urine pH.
    b. Vitamin K is the antagonist for oral anticoagulants. It does not alter urine pH and is not useful in other types of overdoses.
    d. Sodium bicarbonate is given to alkalinize the urine.

12

Ophthalmic, Otic, and Dermatologic Drugs

OVERVIEW

I. Antiglaucoma agents
A. Miotics
B. Beta-blockers
C. Nursing diagnoses
D. Nursing implementation factors
E. Nursing evaluations

II. Adrenergic and anticholinergic mydriatic and cycloplegic agents
A. Adrenergic mydriatic and cycloplegic agents
B. Anticholinergic mydriatic and cycloplegic agents
C. Nursing diagnoses
D. Nursing implementation factors
E. Nursing evaluations

III. Anti-infective and anti-inflammatory agents for the eye
A. Anti-infective agents
B. Anti-inflammatory agents
C. Nursing diagnoses
D. Nursing implementation factors
E. Nursing evaluations

IV. Local and topical anesthetics
A. Examples
B. Use/mechanism of action
C. Adverse effects
D. Contraindications
E. Precautions
F. Drug interactions
G. Nursing diagnoses
H. Nursing implementation factors
I. Nursing evaluations

V. Other topical and dermatologic preparations
A. Examples
B. Use/mechanism of action
C. Adverse effects
D. Contraindications
E. Precautions
F. Drug interactions
G. Nursing diagnoses
H. Nursing implementation factors
I. Nursing evaluations

VI. Ear medications
A. Examples
B. Use/mechanism of action
C. Adverse effects
D. Contraindications
E. Precautions
F. Drug interactions
G. Nursing diagnoses
H. Nursing implementation factors
I. Nursing evaluations

NURSING HIGHLIGHTS

1. Because clients often consider topical medications to be free from risk, nurse should warn them when systemic effects are possible and stress that overuse will cause adverse effects.
2. Nurse should reassure client who experiences a body image disturbance because of minor eye or skin disease that the condition will resolve with proper care.
3. Nurse should stress to glaucoma clients that their medication controls the disorder but does not cure it and must be taken for life.

GLOSSARY

aqueous humor—the fluid produced in the eye that fills the spaces in front of the lens and its attachments

canthus—the angle at either end of the fissure between the eyelids

cycloplegic drug—an agent that paralyzes the ciliary muscle of the eye

keratolytic drug—an agent that softens scales, loosens the stratum corneum, and causes peeling or shedding of the skin; also called a desquamating agent

miotic drug—an agent that causes the pupil to constrict

mydriatic drug—an agent that causes the pupil to dilate

pediculide—an agent that destroys lice

scabicide—an agent that destroys the itch mite, *Sarcoptes scabiei*, the insect that causes scabies

ENHANCED OUTLINE

See text pages
_____

I. Antiglaucoma agents

A. Miotics
   1. Examples: demecarium (Humorsol), echothiophate (Phospholine), isoflurophate (Floropryl), physostigmine (Eserine), pilocarpine (Pilocar)
   2. Use/mechanism of action: treat glaucoma by improving aqueous outflow from inner chamber of eye
   3. Adverse effects: blurred vision, eye and brow pain; gastrointestinal (GI) upset, bronchial constriction and spasm with systemic absorption
   4. Contraindications: history of retinal detachment, known hypersensitivity
   5. Precautions: corneal abrasions
   6. Drug interactions
      a) Echothiophate, isoflurophate, or physostigmine with succinylcholine: respiratory or cardiovascular collapse

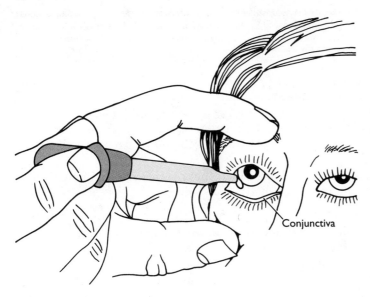

Figure 12–1
Instillation of Eye Drops

        b) Pilocarpine with carbachol: additive effects
        c) Pilocarpine with phenylephrine: decreased mydriasis induced by phenylephrine

B. Beta-blockers
    1. Examples: betaxolol (Betoptic), levobunolol (Betagan), timolol (Timoptic)
    2. Use/mechanism of action: treat glaucoma by lowering intraocular pressure and reducing or blocking aqueous humor formation
    3. Adverse effects: headache, fatigue; bradycardia and bronchospasm with systemic timolol absorption
    4. Contraindications: bronchial asthma, severe chronic obstructive pulmonary disease, known hypersensitivity
    5. Precautions: pregnancy, lactation, cerebral vascular insufficiency
    6. Drug interactions: increased ocular and systemic effects with timolol and oral beta blockers

C. Nursing diagnoses
    1. Sensory-perceptual alterations: visual related to adverse ocular effects of miotic agent and medical condition
    2. Anxiety related to possible decrease or loss of vision
    3. Potential for injury related to concurrent use of local and systemic beta-blocker

D. Nursing implementation factors
    1. Administration procedures
        a) Minimize systemic absorption by applying digital pressure over punctum at inner canthus for 2–3 minutes after instillation.
        b) Administer mild analgesic if client complains of headache.

2. Daily monitoring and measurements
   a) Monitor client receiving miotic agent for signs of bronchial constriction or spasm and pulmonary edema.
   b) Monitor heart rate to detect bradycardia in client receiving beta-blocker.
3. Points for client teaching: Warn client that miotic agents will blur vision and should ideally be instilled at bedtime.

E. Nursing evaluations
   1. Client takes miotic at bedtime to minimize inconvenience and decreased safety of blurred vision.
   2. Client verbalizes concerns.
   3. Client has been taught to minimize systemic absorption by proper drug administration.

See text pages

II. Adrenergic and anticholinergic mydriatic and cycloplegic agents

A. Adrenergic mydriatic and cycloplegic agents
   1. Examples: atropine (Atropisol); dipevefrin (Propine); epinephrine (Epifrin, Glaucon); epinephryl (Epinal); phenylephrine (Neo-Synephrine)
   2. Use/mechanism of action: treat wide-angle glaucoma and glaucoma secondary to uveitis, produce mydriasis for ocular examination, and relieve congestion and hyperemia by contracting the radial or dilator muscle of the eye, constricting conjunctival blood vessels, relaxing ciliary muscle, and decreasing intraocular pressure
   3. Adverse effects (unusual): tachycardia, hypertension
   4. Contraindications: narrow-angle glaucoma or abraded cornea
   5. Precautions: cardiovascular disease
   6. Drug interactions: potentiation of adrenergic pressor effects with tricyclic antidepressants; exaggerated adrenergic effects with MAO (monoamine oxidase) inhibitors

B. Anticholinergic mydriatic and cycloplegic agents
   1. Examples: cyclopentolate (Cyclogyl), homatropine (Homatrocel Ophthalmic), scopolamine (Isopto Hyoscine), tropicamide (Mydriacyl)
   2. Use/mechanism of action: relieve ocular pain caused by uveitis, keratitis, and eye surgery; relax ciliary muscle for accurate measurement of refractive errors by blocking acetylcholine stimulation of sphincter muscle of iris and accommodative muscle of ciliary body
   3. Adverse effects: stinging, red eye, eye irritation, increased intraocular pressure, allergic lid reactions (with local use); sweat inhibition, flushing, dry mouth, fever, delirium, convulsions, tachycardia, ataxia, hallucinations, behavioral problems, respiratory depression, coma (with systemic absorption)

4. Contraindications: known or suspected closed-angle glaucoma
5. Precautions: pregnancy, infancy, spastic paralysis or brain damage in child
6. Drug interactions: none significant

C. Nursing diagnoses
   1. Sensory-perceptual alterations: visual related to adverse ocular effects
   2. Pain related to stinging sensation on application
   3. Potential for injury related to reduced vision

D. Nursing implementation factors
   1. Administration procedures
      a) Minimize systemic absorption by applying digital pressure over punctum at inner canthus for 2–3 minutes after eye drop instillation.
      b) To instill drops, have client look upward, then pull down lower lid and instill prescribed number of drops.
   2. Daily monitoring and measurements
      a) Inspect eyes regularly for irritation, dryness, conjunctivitis, and contact dermatitis.
      b) Observe client for systemic adverse reactions.
   3. Points for client teaching
      a) Warn client that eye irritation, blurred vision, and burning or stinging may occur when drug is instilled.
      b) Show client how to instill drops and advise him/her not to touch dropper to eye or other surface.

E. Nursing evaluations
   1. Client uses drug at bedtime to minimize inconvenience of blurred vision.
   2. Client's eye pain is relieved.
   3. Client maintains activity appropriate to level of vision.

III. Anti-infective and anti-inflammatory agents for the eye

See text pages

_____

A. Anti-infective agents
   1. Examples: bacitracin (AK-Tracin), boric acid (Blinx), chloramphenicol (Chloromycetin Ophthalmic), chlortetracycline (Aureomycin), erythromycin (Ilotycin Ophthalmic), gentamicin (Garamycin), idoxuridine (Herplex), natamycin (Natacyn), polymyxin B (Neosporin Ophthalmic), sulfacetamide (Bleph-10), tetracycline (Achromycin Ophthalmic), tobramycin (Tobrex), trifluridine (Viroptic Ophthalmic Solution), vidarabine (Vira-A Ophthalmic)
   2. Use/mechanism of action: treat bacterial or viral eye infections by penetrating the cornea and conjunctiva (bacitracin, polymyxin B); penetrating the cornea, conjunctiva, and aqueous humor (chloramphenicol, tobramycin); and penetrating corneal abrasions but not the intact cornea (gentamicin, tetracyclines)
   3. Adverse effects: hypersensitivity to sulfonamides, secondary eye infections (with prolonged use), aplastic anemia, Stevens-Johnson syndrome

    4. Contraindications: corneal abrasions, known hypersensitivity

    5. Precautions: none significant

    6. Drug interactions: inactivation of bacitracin when used with silver nitrate; decreased efficacy of sulfacetamide when used with local anesthetic

B. Anti-inflammatory agents

    1. Examples: fluorometholone (Fluor-Op, FML); medrysone (HMS Liquifilm Ophthalmic); prednisolone (Econopred, Pred Forte)

    2. Use/mechanism of action: reduce inflammation by decreasing local leukocyte infiltration

    3. Adverse effects: increased intraocular pressure, corneal thinning or ulcerations, increased susceptibility to corneal infection; worsening glaucoma, cataracts, reduced acuity, optic nerve damage with long-term use; adrenal suppression (with long-term use of suspensions)

    4. Contraindications: acute, untreated eye infection; viral disease of cornea or conjunctiva

    5. Precautions: corneal abrasions

    6. Drug interactions: none significant

C. Nursing diagnoses

    1. Altered sensory perception: visual related to ocular disorder

    2. Potential for injury related to altered vision

D. Nursing implementation factors

    1. Administration procedures: Administer sulfacetamide 30–60 minutes after local anesthetic to avoid drug interaction.

    2. Daily monitoring and measurements

      a) Check client's eyes regularly for signs of infection during anti-inflammatory therapy.

      b) Ascertain that regular ocular examinations are scheduled while client is receiving anti-inflammatory therapy.

    3. Points for client teaching

      a) Instruct client to shake suspension of anti-inflammatory agent thoroughly before instillation.

      b) Show client how to apply pressure on punctum at inner canthus to minimize systemic absorption.

      c) Stress importance of regular eye examinations.

      d) Teach client good hygiene to prevent spread of infection (see Client Teaching Checklist, "Eye Medications").

E. Nursing evaluations

    1. Client experiences an improvement in eye disorder.

    2. Client avoids injury related to vision disorder.

IV. Local and topical anesthetics

See text pages

A. Examples
1. Local anesthetics: bupivacaine (Marcaine), chloroprocaine (Nesacaine), etidocaine (Duranest), lidocaine (Xylocaine), mepivacaine (Carbocaine), prilocaine (Citanest), procaine (Novocain), propoxycaine (Ravocaine), tetracaine (Pontocaine)
2. Topical anesthetics: benzocaine (Anbesol), benzyl alcohol, butacaine, butamben (Butesin), dibucaine (Nupercainal), dyclonine (Dyclone), lidocaine (Xylocaine), tetracaine (Pontocaine)

B. Use/mechanism of action: prevent or relieve pain by blocking transmission of impulses across nerve cell membranes or interfering with pain perception by counterirritation of nerve (benzyl alcohol)

C. Adverse effects (occurring with overdose or improper injection techniques with local anesthetics): anxiety, nervousness, disorientation, tremor, confusion, shivering, seizures, followed by central nervous system (CNS) depression; myocardial depression, bradycardia, cardiac arrhythmias, hypotension, cardiovascular collapse, cardiac arrest with high plasma levels; contact dermatitis, stromal edema

D. Contraindications: septicemia, severe hypertension, skin disease

E. Precautions: cardiovascular disease, pregnancy, shock, severe anemia

F. Drug interactions: incompatibility of tetracaine with mercury or silver salts often found in ophthalmic products; cardiac arrhythmias when etidocaine, mepivacaine, or bupivacaine is used with enflurane and related inhalation anesthetics

G. Nursing diagnoses
1. Pain related to underlying disorder
2. Anxiety related to pain

H. Nursing implementation factors
1. Administration procedures
   a) Discard partially used vials of anesthetics that do not contain preservatives.

b) Administer topical lidocaine cautiously to client with large areas of broken skin or mucous membranes.
c) Use lowest dose of topical anesthetic needed to relieve pain.
2. Daily monitoring and measurements
a) In pregnant client, monitor fetus for bradycardia or acidosis.
b) Observe extremity that has been anesthetized for peripheral pulse, color, and temperature.
3. Points for client teaching
a) Caution client to protect numb areas until sensation returns.
b) Warn client to avoid getting topical anesthetic into eyes.
I. Nursing evaluations
1. Area is successfully anesthetized and client's pain is relieved.
2. Client's anxiety is relieved.

See text pages
_____

V. Other topical and dermatologic preparations

A. Examples
1. Antimycotic (antifungal) agents: amphotericin B (Fungizone), nystatin (Mycostatin)
2. Antibacterial agents: bacitracin (Baciguent), chloramphenicol (Chloromycetin), clindamycin (Cleocin T)
3. Scabicides and pediculicides: benzyl benzoate; lindane (Scabene, Kwell)
4. Keratolytics and caustics: anthralin (Anthra-Derm), cantharidin (Cantharone), podophyllum (Pod-Ben-25), resorcinol, silver nitrate
5. Corticosteroids: fluticasone (Cutivate), mometasone (Elocon)
6. Antiseptics and disinfectants: chlorhexidine (Hibiclens), ethyl alcohol, isopropyl alcohol, hexachlorophene (pHisoHex), hydrogen peroxide, iodine

B. Use/mechanism of action: reduce inflammation, prevent infection of minor wounds, and treat various skin conditions, including fungal and bacterial infections, scabies, pediculosis, dermatitis from various causes, warts and other benign growths, hyperkeratotic conditions such as psoriasis, by a wide range of mechanisms, including killing bacteria, viruses, fungi, and parasitic worms

C. Adverse effects: hypersensitivity reactions, such as rashes

D. Contraindications: known hypersensitivity

E. Precautions: large areas of broken skin

F. Drug interactions: few significant

G. Nursing diagnoses
1. Potential for impaired skin integrity related to rash
2. Body image disturbance related to skin lesions

H. Nursing implementation factors
   1. Administration procedures
      a) Ensure that any required laboratory specimens are obtained before the start of therapy.
      b) Follow administration procedures, noting whether medication should be applied sparingly or liberally.
   2. Daily monitoring and measurements
      a) Observe client for therapeutic and hypersensitivity responses.
      b) Check client using topical corticosteroids for signs of bacterial, fungal, or viral overgrowth.
   3. Points for client teaching
      a) Warn client not to get medication into mouth or eyes.
      b) Remind client to keep all medications away from children and to follow instructions about appropriate temperature range for storing medication.
      c) Caution client to complete entire course of treatment.

I. Nursing evaluations
   1. Client's dermatologic problem is relieved by prescribed agent.
   2. Client understands that the skin condition can be controlled with good compliance and has a positive attitude.

VI. Ear medications

See text pages
_____

A. Examples
   1. Anti-infective agents: acetic acid (Domeboro Otic), boric acid (Ear-Dry), chloramphenicol (Chloromycetin Otic), colistin, polymyxin B
   2. Anti-inflammatory agents: dexamethasone (AK-Dex), hydrocortisone
   3. Local anesthetics: benzocaine (Americaine Otic)
   4. Ceruminolytic agents: carbamide (Debrox), triethanolamine (Cerumenex)

B. Use/mechanism of action: treat infection and inflammation by mechanisms discussed in Chapter 3, section II,B,2 and in Chapter 9, sections I,B; II,B; and III,B; relieve pain by blocking transmission of impulses across nerve cell membranes; soften cerumen (earwax) by emulsification

C. Adverse effects
   1. Anti-infective agents: superinfections
   2. Anti-inflammatory agents: local burning and stinging; masked otic infection
   3. Local anesthetics: irritation, pruritus, edema, masked otic infection, hypersensitivity (all with benzocaine)
   4. Ceruminolytic agents: mild erythema, pruritus

D. Contraindications: perforated tympanic membrane (all agents), acute otic infection (anti-inflammatory agents)

E. Precautions: none significant

F. Drug interactions: none significant

G. Nursing diagnoses
   1. Pain related to ear disorder
   2. Hyperthermia related to ear infection

H. Nursing implementation factors
   1. Administration procedures
      a) Warm ear drops to room temperature before instillation by rolling bottle in palms of hands.
      b) To administer medication to adult, position client with affected ear up, then pull top of ear up and back.
      c) To administer medication to child younger than 4 years old, position client with affected ear up, then pull lobe of ear down and back gently.
      d) Have client remain on unaffected side for 20 minutes after administration to prevent medicine from coming out of ear.
   2. Daily monitoring and measurements: Check ear regularly.
   3. Points for client teaching
      a) Caution client to notify physician or nurse immediately if hearing acuity decreases or he/she experiences tinnitus, dizziness, or unsteady gait while using an anti-infective or local anesthetic.
      b) Advise client not to wash ear dropper after use.

I. Nursing evaluations
   1. Client's ear disorder improves and pain is relieved.
   2. Client's temperature returns to normal.

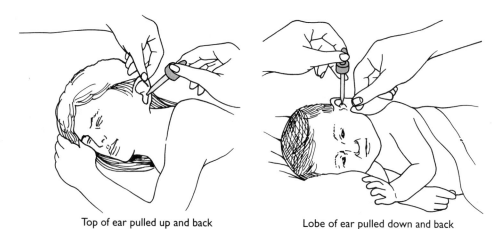

Top of ear pulled up and back   Lobe of ear pulled down and back

Figure 12–2
Ear Drop Administration in Children and Adults

1. Phenylephrine hydrochloride (Neo-Synephrine) eye drops have been administered to Mr. Terrell for their mydriatic effect. The nurse recognizes that the drops are having their intended effect when his pupils:

   a. Are constricted.
   b. Are dilated.
   c. Do not respond to light.
   d. Do not accommodate for near vision.

2. When systemic absorption of physostigmine (Eserine) eye drops occurs, which of the following side effects can be expected?

   a. Bradycardia
   b. Tachycardia
   c. Orthostatic hypotension
   d. Dyspnea

3. The client who is receiving pilocarpine (Isopto Carpine) eye drops to treat glaucoma should be told to:

   a. Wear dark glasses in brightly lit environments.
   b. Discontinue the drops if brow or eyelid pain occurs.
   c. Instill the drops before beginning daily activities.
   d. Notify the physician if dark pigmentation appears around the iris.

4. To minimize systemic absorption of medications applied topically to the eye, the nurse should:

   a. Instill the drops at the outer canthus of the affected eye.
   b. Turn the client's head so outer canthus of affected eye is lower than inner canthus.
   c. Put pressure on inner canthus of affected eye for 2–3 minutes after instilling medication.
   d. Apply the drops under the upper lid and have the client blink several times.

5. The client who is receiving betaxolol hydrochloride (Betoptic) eye drops to reduce intraocular pressure must be monitored for which adverse effect?

   a. Decreased visual acuity
   b. Palpitations
   c. Bradycardia
   d. Inequality of pupil size

6. Tyrone Johnson receives an injection of lidocaine (Xylocaine) to anesthetize his arm before having a laceration sutured. One minute after the injection he reports that his arm feels hot. The nurse should:

   a. Prepare to administer epinephrine to control an allergic reaction.
   b. Raise the affected arm above the level of his heart.
   c. Apply cold compresses proximal to the wound.
   d. Reassure him that this is a sign the anesthetic is taking effect.

7. Martha Brady is using benzocaine (Solarcaine) to control pain from a severe sunburn. She should be advised to:

   a. Inspect her skin for rashes before applying the next dose.
   b. Rub the ointment thoroughly into the affected area.
   c. Discontinue use if a stinging sensation occurs when the ointment is applied.
   d. Remove the previous application with rubbing alcohol before applying the next dose.

8. Packing soaked with sodium hypochlorite (Dakin's) solution is ordered to treat Mrs. Arnold's stage III decubitus ulcer. When the old packing is removed, the wound is draining a large amount of yellow pus. The nurse should:

   a. Use a gauze pad soaked with saline to clean away all drainage before applying the new packing.

Ophthalmic, Otic, and Dermatologic Drugs   223

b. Flush the wound with diluted peroxide solution and rinse with saline before packing the wound.

c. Pack dry gauze into the wound, leave it for 30 minutes, then remove it and apply the Dakin's solution–soaked packing.

d. Consult the physician about ordering a different antiseptic solution for the wound packing.

9. The physician orders an occlusive dressing over antibiotic ointment to treat a large laceration on the client's arm. The nurse should cover the area with:

a. A double layer of gauze with all edges taped down.

b. A single gauze pad completely covered with overlapping strips of tape.

c. A gauze pad under a piece of plastic wrap with all edges taped down.

d. A double layer of gauze held in place with several turns of rolled gauze bandage.

10. Mrs. Kelly has been applying desonide (Tridesilon) cream to an area of psoriasis on her elbow for 2 weeks. The area now appears slightly red and Mrs. Kelly reports a stinging sensation. The nurse should:

a. Advise her to use a soft gauze dressing over the desonide cream.

b. Discontinue the desonide cream and notify the physician.

c. Suggest cleaning the lesion with isopropyl alcohol before applying the desonide cream.

d. Consult the physician about increasing the frequency of application of the desonide cream.

11. The client for whom malathion (Prioderm) shampoo is prescribed to treat head lice should be told to:

a. Avoid using a hair dryer after using malathion shampoo.

b. Avoid washing the hair for 24 hours after application.

c. Wrap the head in a towel for 4 hours after applying malathion.

d. Rinse the hair with a dilute vinegar solution after 8 hours.

12. Before administering antibiotic ear drops, the nurse should:

a. Clean the ear canal with a cotton-tipped applicator.

b. Roll the medication bottle between the palms for 30–60 seconds.

c. Gently irrigate the ear canal with warm saline solution.

d. Have the client lie on the affected side for 5 minutes.

ANSWERS

1. Correct answer is b. Mydriasis refers to dilation of the pupil. Adrenergics such as phenylephrine provide mydriasis without cycloplegia.

a. Pupillary constriction describes miosis, the effect of cholinergic drops.

c. Failure to respond to light is not a desired effect of any ocular medication.

d. Lack of accommodation for near vision describes cycloplegia, which is an effect of anticholinergic drops. Anticholinergics also produce mydriasis.

2. Correct answer is d. Systemic effects of cholinergic agents include bronchoconstriction, which produces dyspnea.

a. Bradycardia results from systemic absorption of a beta-adrenergic blocking drug.

b. Tachycardia results from systemic absorption of adrenergic or anticholinergic drops.

c. Orthostatic hypotension is not an anticipated side effect of systemic absorption of any type of eye drops.

3. **Correct answer is a.** Cholinergic drops may cause painful sensitivity to light. Dark glasses will minimize this effect.

   b. Brow or eyelid pain is a common side effect. The drops should be discontinued only if pain becomes severe.
   c. Miotic drops should be instilled at bedtime to minimize safety concerns related to blurred vision.
   d. Cholinergics do not change pigmentation of the iris. Depigmentation of eyelid skin indicates a hypersensitivity reaction in dark-skinned individuals.

4. **Correct answer is c.** Systemic absorption of drops occurs when they drain through the nasolacrimal duct onto nasal mucosa. Pressing the inner canthus blocks the nasolacrimal duct long enough for the drops to be absorbed into the surface of the eye.

   a. There is little space under the lower lid at the outer canthus, so part of the instilled drop would be lost. Since liquids instilled into the eye drain toward the inner canthus, some might still reach the nasolacrimal duct.
   b. With the outer canthus lower than the inner canthus, it would be difficult to instill drops into the eye. The position might also cause medication to drain out of the eye in tears.
   d. It would be difficult to instill drops under the upper lid without contaminating the dropper. Blinking distributes the drops over the surface of the eye but does not prevent drainage into the nasolacrimal duct.

5. **Correct answer is c.** Beta-adrenergic blocking agents commonly cause bradycardia. Systemic absorption of eye drops is sufficient to produce bradycardia.

   a. Decreased visual acuity might indicate worsening of glaucoma. It is not an adverse effect of the drug.
   b. Palpitations are seen with adrenergic or anticholinergic medications, not with beta-blockers.

   d. Unequal pupil size is a common variation among people without any pathology. It is not an effect of beta-blocking drugs. Significant or new differences in pupil size reflect cranial nerve pathology.

6. **Correct answer is d.** As local anesthetics take effect, cold sensation is lost first. This produces a transient sensation of warmth before heat sensation is lost.

   a. A feeling of hotness is not a sign of an allergic reaction. Edema, rash, or respiratory symptoms are signs of allergy.
   b. Raising the arm is contraindicated, since it would facilitate venous drainage, carrying more of the local anesthetic into systemic circulation.
   c. While a cold compress might be offered as a comfort measure under other circumstances, it is irrelevant in this case. Heat sensation will be lost quickly, relieving the hot feeling.

7. **Correct answer is a.** Rash is a sign of allergy to local anesthetics. Due to the anesthetic, pain or itching may be absent, so visual checks are important.

   b. A thin layer of benzocaine should be applied with gentle strokes. Rubbing may damage the burned tissues.
   c. A mild stinging sensation when ointment is first applied is not unusual. If there is no rash or open area, this is not a cause for concern.
   d. Previously applied medication should be removed with mild soap and water. Alcohol is a drying agent, which predisposes the skin to cracks and breaks that increase the risk of infection.

8. **Correct answer is d.** Dakin's solution, which is indicated to deodorize and dissolve necrotic tissue, is inactivated by purulent drainage.

   a. While cleaning with a saline-soaked gauze pad would be appropriate before dressing the wound, it ignores the central concern, that the medication will be inactivated by the drainage.

b. Peroxide solutions should not be used without physician's orders. Peroxide's foaming action can damage healing tissue or cause air emboli.

c. Dry gauze would offer no antiseptic action, permitting bacterial growth under the packing. The presence of pus indicates bacterial contamination of the wound.

9. **Correct answer is c.** This provides a completely occlusive dressing.

   a. Even a double layer of gauze is not occlusive.

   b. Although a gauze pad that is covered with strips of tape is more occlusive than gauze alone, tape is not impermeable to moisture.

   d. A double layer of gauze held in place with rolled gauze bandage would keep tape from contacting the skin, preventing skin stripping when the dressing is changed, but it is not occlusive.

10. **Correct answer is b.** Because corticosteroids suppress the inflammatory response, the risk of infection is increased. Because usual signs of infection, such as redness, swelling, pain, and drainage, are suppressed by corticosteroids, even mild symptoms should be investigated. The suppressed inflammatory response will permit any existing infection to worsen rapidly.

    a. A soft gauze dressing might be indicated to protect clothing or avoid irritating the lesion, but any inflammatory symptoms should be investigated first. Infection can spread rapidly under a dressing.

c. The drying effects of alcohol may lead to cracking of the skin. Open areas increase the risk of infection or systemic drug absorption.

d. A dosage increase is not appropriate until the possibility of infection has been investigated.

11. **Correct answer is a.** Malathion is flammable, so use of any electrical appliance or open flame near the treated hair must be avoided. The hair should be allowed to air-dry.

    b. The hair should be washed and combed in 8–12 hours to remove the malathion and dead lice.

    c. Wrapping the head in a towel is unnecessary and might promote systemic absorption of malathion.

    d. The hair should be washed with a mild shampoo to remove the malathion. Vinegar would have no useful effect and its acid content might worsen any irritation caused by the malathion.

12. **Correct answer is b.** To prevent vertigo or nausea, ear drops should be warmed before administration.

    a. Applicators should never be inserted into the ear canal. This could force infectious material deeper into the canal or puncture the tympanic membrane.

    c. The ear should not be irrigated unless ordered by the physician. Irrigation solution could carry infectious material to uninfected parts of the ear.

    d. Lying on the affected side might promote drainage of infectious material out of the ear, but 5 minutes is probably an inadequate time period for such drainage to occur.

Nursing Pharmacology Comprehensive Review Questions

1. For which of the following clients should the nurse anticipate problems with biotransformation of drugs?

   a. A 12-year-old with an ear infection
   b. A 35-year-old asthmatic
   c. An 18-year-old with pyelonephritis
   d. A 57-year-old with congestive heart failure

2. When a drug has a low therapeutic index, the nurse can expect that:

   a. Other drugs will need to be given to potentiate its therapeutic effect.
   b. The drug will have few serious side effects.
   c. The potential for toxicity will be great.
   d. Low doses of the drug will produce side effects.

3. An appropriate site for administration of subcutaneous heparin is:

   a. The anterior surface of the upper arm.
   b. The area above the scapula.
   c. 1 inch above the umbilicus.
   d. The inner surface of the thigh.

4. Mrs. Clifford is breastfeeding her 4-week-old son. When she develops a urinary tract infection, her physician prescribes ampicillin and tells her she does not have to stop breastfeeding. Which advice should the nurse give Mrs. Clifford?

   a. Take the drug every 6 hours, regardless of the feeding schedule.
   b. Schedule the drug doses a half hour before feedings.
   c. Take the drug right after a feeding.
   d. Pump both breasts and discard the milk 1 hour after taking the drug.

5. Side effects caused by central nervous system (CNS) depression or stimulation occur only with drugs that reach brain tissue. The nurse should anticipate CNS side effects with drugs that are:

   a. Water soluble.
   b. Lipid soluble.
   c. Acidic.
   d. Alkaline.

6. An appropriate nursing diagnosis for a client taking cyclobenzaprine (Flexeril) for lower-back strain is:

   a. Sleep pattern disturbance related to CNS stimulation.
   b. Altered oral mucous membranes related to excretion of drug metabolites in saliva.
   c. High risk for injury related to impaired judgment.
   d. Urinary frequency related to cholinergic side effects.

7. The client taking clozapine (Clozaril) to control schizophrenic symptoms must have frequent monitoring of:

   a. White blood cell count (WBC).
   b. Hemoglobin and hematocrit.
   c. Blood urea nitrogen (BUN) and creatinine.
   d. Liver enzymes.

8. The nurse is most likely to recognize early signs of tardive dyskinesia secondary to antipsychotic drugs by observing the client:

   a. Holding arms straight forward and parallel to the floor.
   b. Sticking the tongue out.
   c. Walking without assistance.
   d. Touching the nose with the eyes closed.

9. The client who will be taking oral anticoagulants at home should be taught to make which dietary modification?

   a. Avoid caffeine.
   b. Eat more bananas, raisins, and potatoes.
   c. Reduce intake of green leafy vegetables.
   d. Increase intake of dairy products.

10. Mrs. D'Amico has difficulty swallowing pills. Her iron deficiency anemia is being treated with a liquid iron preparation. She should be taught to:

    a. Mix the liquid iron in milk.
    b. Drink the liquid iron through a straw.
    c. Take the iron with meals.
    d. Take an antacid if iron causes GI distress.

11. Joshua Wilson has bronchitis and complains that his cough keeps him awake and makes his ribs ache. Benzonatate (Tessalon) is prescribed. Mr. Wilson asks, "Wouldn't codeine be better for stopping this cough? It's really severe." The nurse should tell Mr. Wilson that:

    a. Benzonatate has the same effects as codeine.
    b. Benzonatate is slightly less effective but will not cause drowsiness.
    c. Benzonatate is equally effective but will not cause drowsiness.
    d. Benzonatate has the same effects as codeine without causing physical dependence.

12. Humidification is required when nasal oxygen is given at flow rates greater than:

    a. 2 l/min.
    b. 4 l/min.
    c. 6 l/min.
    d. 8 l/min.

13. The best method for administering an antacid suspension to prevent stress ulcers is to:

    a. Have the client drink 8 oz of water, then the antacid.
    b. Have the client take the antacid, then drink 8 oz of water.
    c. Mix the antacid in 4 oz of water before administering.
    d. Have the client avoid drinking within 30 minutes of taking the antacid.

14. Elisa Barr is taking chlorpromazine (Thorazine) 100 mg by rectal suppository every 8 hours to control nausea due to cancer chemotherapy. She should be taught to:

    a. Eat a low-residue diet while using chlorpromazine.
    b. Get up slowly, pausing in a sitting position before standing.
    c. Empty her bladder on a regular schedule to avoid incontinence.
    d. Use higher-wattage bulbs in lamps to compensate for pupil constriction.

15. Oxytocin (Pitocin) has been administered to Mrs. Brady to induce labor. As delivery approaches, saddle-block anesthesia is given. The nurse needs to monitor for which complication of this combination?

    a. Hypertensive crisis
    b. Respiratory depression
    c. Oversedation of the infant
    d. Postpartum hemorrhage

16. To prevent hypotension during IV infusion of ritodrine (Yutopar) to stop preterm labor, the nurse should position the client:

    a. On her left side.
    b. In a high Fowler's position.
    c. In Trendelenburg's position.
    d. On her right side.

17. Mrs. Carter, 27 years old, is being treated for an upper respiratory infection with ampicillin (Omnipen). The nurse should inform her that:

    a. Ampicillin should be taken with food.
    b. She should avoid all alcohol-containing beverages and medications.
    c. She should wear protective clothing and use an SPF-15 sunscreen when outside.
    d. If she takes oral contraceptives she will need to use an additional contraceptive method.

18. Aspirin should not be administered to:

   a. Clients with impaired liver function.

   b. Clients receiving urinary acidifying agents.

   c. Children with viral infections.

   d. Elderly clients with rheumatoid arthritis.

19. Mrs. Adams is receiving cyclophosphamide (Cytoxan) to treat lymphocytic leukemia. To prevent hemorrhagic cystitis, the nurse should expect to:

   a. Premedicate Mrs. Adams with sodium bicarbonate.

   b. Premedicate Mrs. Adams with ascorbic acid.

   c. Administer a liter of IV saline solution before the cyclophosphamide.

   d. Administer the cyclophosphamide at bedtime.

20. Before administering influenza virus vaccine (Fluogen), the nurse should ask whether the client is allergic to:

   a. Penicillin.

   b. Eggs.

   c. Horse serum.

   d. Iodine.

21. Niacin should not be administered to the client who has:

   a. Renal insufficiency.

   b. Peptic ulcer.

   c. Congestive heart failure.

   d. Rheumatoid arthritis.

22. Mr. Arters, who takes levodopa for Parkinson's disease, tells the nurse that he plans to start taking a multivitamin. The nurse should suggest that he use a preparation that does not contain:

   a. Vitamin D.

   b. Iron.

   c. Pyridoxine (vitamin B_6).

   d. Zinc.

23. An appropriate nursing diagnosis to describe side effects of iodine therapy for treating goiter is:

   a. Altered nutrition, less than body requirements, related to altered taste sensation.

   b. Constipation related to slowed peristalsis.

   c. Fluid volume deficit related to osmotic diuresis.

   d. Hypothermia related to depression of the hypothalamus.

24. To detect drug toxicity, the nurse should monitor the client receiving polymyxin B ear drops for an ear infection for:

   a. Jaundice.

   b. Dyspnea.

   c. Unsteady gait.

   d. Irregular pulse.

25. To administer ear drops to an 8-year-old child, the nurse should:

   a. Pull the pinna of the ear up and back.

   b. Pull the lobe of the ear down and back.

   c. Pull the pinna of the ear outward at a 45° angle to the head.

   d. Not move the ear at all, since the ear of an 8-year-old child is at an intermediate stage of development.

ANSWERS

1. Correct answer is d. Biotransformation of most drugs is a function of the liver. Congestive heart failure decreases circulation through the liver, reducing delivery of the drug to its metabolic sites.

   a. Altered liver function is seen at the extremes of age, but this applies only to infants. By middle childhood the liver should be functioning well. Acute infections do not usually alter liver function.

   b. Respiratory diseases do not usually have a significant impact on liver function or circulation.

   c. Renal disease might alter drug excretion but does not normally impair liver functions, except in the late stages of chronic renal failure.

2. **Correct answer is c.** Therapeutic index (the ratio of toxic dose to therapeutic dose) is used to evaluate a drug's potential toxicity. The nurse must watch for signs of toxicity when the therapeutic index is low.

   a. Since therapeutic index does not provide information about a drug's therapeutic effectiveness, it is not a criterion for prescribing adjunctive drugs.
   b. Since the therapeutic dose of a drug with a low therapeutic index is close to the toxic dose, the likelihood of side effects is, if affected at all, increased.
   d. Therapeutic index does not indicate the size of a safe dose.

3. **Correct answer is b.** The area of subcutaneous fat over the scapula is one of the preferred sites for subcutaneous heparin injection.

   a. The anterior surface of the upper arm is not used for subcutaneous injection because the subcutaneous fat is thinner there. Although the posterior surface of the upper arm is an adequate subcutaneous injection site, it is not used for heparin because frequent muscle action in the area would increase the risk of bleeding at the injection site, causing ecchymoses to form.
   c. The abdomen is one of the preferred sites for heparin, but injections must be given at least 2 inches from the umbilicus.
   d. The inner thigh is not used for injections. The area from midanterior to midlateral thigh is an accepted subcutaneous injection site but is not used for heparin for the reason noted in a.

4. **Correct answer is c.** Taking the medication immediately after a feeding and postponing the next feeding for at least 4 hours minimizes the infant's drug exposure.

   a. Taking the drug every 6 hours would provide consistent plasma levels for the mother but does nothing to minimize the infant's exposure to the drug.
   b. Taking the drug a half hour before feedings would cause plasma levels to peak when the feeding is due, increasing the infant's drug exposure.
   d. Discarding the milk is an unnecessary precaution that might result in inadequate milk for the infant's needs.

5. **Correct answer is b.** To reach brain tissue, a drug must cross the blood-brain barrier. Since only lipid-soluble drugs cross this lipoid barrier, they are the ones expected to cause CNS side effects.

   a. Water-soluble drugs do not penetrate the blood-brain barrier to reach brain tissue.
   c and d. A drug's pH has no effect on whether it crosses the blood-brain barrier.

6. **Correct answer is c.** CNS depressant effects of skeletal muscle relaxants include impaired judgment, slowed motor responses, confusion, and drowsiness. All increase the risk for injuries.

   a. Skeletal muscle relaxants are not CNS stimulants. This nursing diagnosis is appropriate for psychomotor stimulant drugs.
   b. Focus on altered mucous membranes is appropriate for hydantoin anticonvulsants, such as phenytoin. No metabolites of skeletal muscle relaxants are excreted in saliva.
   d. Cyclobenzaprine has anticholinergic side effects that include urinary retention, not frequency.

7. **Correct answer is a.** Potentially fatal agranulocytosis is the major adverse effect of clozapine. During the first 6 months of therapy, the white blood cell count (WBC) is usually monitored weekly, since this reaction most commonly appears in this time period.

   b. Neither anemia nor bleeding is a common side effect of clozapine, so hemoglobin and hematocrit testing is not indicated.
   c. Clozapine is not highly nephrotoxic, so BUN and creatinine do not need frequent monitoring.
   d. Liver enzymes are monitored to detect hepatotoxicity in clients taking phenothiazines. Clozapine does not have the same tendency to damage liver tissue.

8. **Correct answer is b.** Fine wormlike tongue movements are an early sign of tardive dyskinesia. Sticking the tongue out may elicit these movements.

   a. Holding the arms forward is used to elicit asterixis, the flapping tremor of hepatic coma. It is no more effective than any other arm movement for detecting extrapyramidal symptoms.
   c. Gait is most affected by parkinsonism, in which a propulsive shuffling gait is seen.
   d. Touching the nose with closed eyes tests cerebellar function, which is not affected by antipsychotics. Abnormal movements due to antipsychotics originate in the extrapyramidal system.

9. **Correct answer is c.** Green leafy vegetables are high in vitamin K, which antagonizes the action of oral anticoagulants.

   a. Although avoiding caffeine may be a desirable action for the cardiac client, it is not specifically indicated when oral anticoagulants are used.
   b. Eating bananas, raisins, and potatoes increases potassium intake. However, potassium is not affected by oral anticoagulants. This action is indicated for clients taking thiazide or loop diuretics.
   d. Increased intake of dairy products increases calcium. Although calcium is one factor in effective clotting, it is not the factor affected by oral anticoagulants.

10. **Correct answer is b.** Liquid iron preparations can stain the teeth. Using a straw minimizes contact of the medication with the teeth.

    a. Milk inhibits iron absorption and should not be taken with it.
    c. For maximum absorption, iron should be taken on an empty stomach. GI distress may be minimized by taking it with a full glass of water.
    d. Antacids bind iron in the GI tract, decreasing free iron available for absorption.

11. **Correct answer is d.** Benzonatate is an equally effective antitussive and does cause

sedation, but it does not have the same potential for physical dependence as codeine.

   a. Since the potential for physical dependence is not the same, it would be inaccurate to say that benzonatate has the same effects as codeine.
   b. Benzonatate does cause drowsiness, and its antitussive effect is equal to that of codeine.
   c. Benzonatate does cause drowsiness.

12. **Correct answer is b.** Nasal oxygen is very drying to nasal and oral mucosa at flow rates above 4 l/min.

   a. Humidification is not required for low-flow oxygen, although it may be used as a comfort measure. Adequate fluid intake and frequent mouth care should be sufficient to keep mucosa moist.
   c and d. High-flow oxygen does require humidification.

13. **Correct answer is b.** Taking fluid after the antacid flushes the medication through the esophagus and into the stomach, where it has its therapeutic effect. A full 8-oz glass of fluid provides sufficient water to distribute the antacid throughout the stomach, promoting acid neutralization throughout the gastric contents.

   a. Eating a low-residue diet would not flush the medication through the esophagus and into the stomach.
   c. If medication is mixed in fluid and the client fails to drink the full amount, the nurse has no way to know how much of the medication was actually ingested. Since clients may find the taste unpleasant, they may have difficulty consuming the entire 4 oz.
   d. Because not drinking fluids for 30 minutes would leave a significant portion coating the esophagus, it might be an appropriate means of administration for reflux esophagitis. However, it would not provide optimal acid neutralization to prevent stress ulcers.

14. **Correct answer is b.** Orthostatic hypotension is a common side effect of phenothiazines, especially chlorpromazine. Rising slowly and resting briefly in a sitting position before standing up will help prevent dizziness or syncope.

   a. Constipation is a potential side effect of phenothiazines. Dietary fiber should be increased.
   c. Urinary retention is a common side effect of phenothiazines. Incontinence is not a major concern.
   d. Phenothiazines have anticholinergic effects, including pupil dilation. Increased light levels are not needed and may even cause discomfort due to the client's heightened sensitivity to bright light.

15. **Correct answer is a.** Hypertensive crisis, evidenced by sudden increase in blood pressure, severe headache, or epistaxis, may occur when local or regional anesthesia is given with oxytocin.

   b. Local anesthesia does not produce respiratory depression, either alone or in combination with oxytocin.
   c. Neither oxytocin nor local anesthetics should have sedating effects on the infant. Since local anesthetics are not rapidly absorbed into maternal systemic circulation, they should not reach the fetus before delivery. Oxytocin speeds the progress of labor, further reducing the risk.
   d. Oxytocin stimulates uterine contraction, reducing the risk of postpartum bleeding.

16. **Correct answer is a.** Lying on the left side prevents the abdominal organs from exerting pressure on the inferior vena cava, promoting adequate blood return to the heart. This helps to prevent hypotension.

   b. The postural effects of sitting are likely to decrease blood pressure further.
   c. Having the head lowered allows the abdominal organs to prevent full lung expansion, resulting in decreased oxygenation. This would counteract any benefit of preventing hypotension.

   d. Lying on the right side permits the abdominal organs to press on the inferior vena cava, reducing blood return to the heart.

17. **Correct answer is d.** Ampicillin decreases the efficacy of oral contraceptives. An additional contraceptive method should be used during the entire cycle in which ampicillin is taken, since ovulation may occur.

   a. Ampicillin, like all penicillins, achieves the most effective drug levels when taken on an empty stomach.
   b. Alcohol intolerance is seen with certain cephalosporins but is not a major concern with penicillins.
   c. Photosensitivity is not a major concern with penicillins. These are appropriate protective measures for the client taking tetracyclines.

18. **Correct answer is c.** A correlation has been found between the occurrence of Reye's syndrome following viral illnesses and the use of aspirin. Since alternative medications are available, the risk of using aspirin is not justified.

   a. Impaired liver function would be a concern with acetaminophen (Tylenol), which can be hepatotoxic in large doses or with prolonged use. Aspirin does not have this effect.
   b. Aspirin is excreted more rapidly in acid urine, so its effect may be diminished. Acid urine is not a contraindication for aspirin.
   d. Aspirin is actually the drug of choice to treat rheumatoid arthritis.

19. **Correct answer is c.** Forcing fluids is usually adequate to prevent hemorrhagic cystitis due to cyclophosphamide. Since antineoplastic drugs may cause nausea and vomiting, IV fluids may be necessary to hydrate the client well enough to empty the metabolites from the bladder rapidly.

   a and b. Altering urinary pH has no effect on the risk of hemorrhagic cystitis. Sodium bicarbonate alkalinizes the urine, and ascorbic acid acidifies it. Neither is used to premedicate before cyclophosphamide.

d. Cyclophosphamide should be given early in the day. Urine remains longer in the bladder overnight, which prolongs contact of metabolites with the bladder lining, increasing the risk of cystitis.

20. **Correct answer is b.** The virus used to produce the vaccine is incubated in eggs, and the vaccine may contain some egg yolk protein. Accordingly, it should not be administered to clients allergic to eggs.

    a. Penicillin allergy is not a contraindication to influenza vaccine. Neomycin or streptomycin is used to attenuate the virus in some vaccines, such as measles-mumps-rubella, so allergies to these antibiotics may be significant.
    c. Horse serum is used to produce some immune serums, such as antirabies serum. It is not used for vaccines.
    d. Iodine is not used in the preparation of vaccines. Iodine allergy is significant in clients who will be receiving dyes for diagnostic x-rays.

21. **Correct answer is b.** Niacin stimulates histamine release, which increases gastric secretion. This can exacerbate peptic ulcers.

    a. Renal insufficiency is not a contraindication to niacin therapy.
    c. Congestive heart failure is not a contraindication to niacin therapy. Niacin is sometimes used to treat cardiovascular disease because of its lipid-lowering effects.
    d. Rheumatoid arthritis is not a contraindication for niacin. Gouty arthritis is an indication for cautious use, since niacin can elevate uric acid levels.

22. **Correct answer is c.** Pyridoxine speeds the metabolism of levodopa and may decrease its effect. Pyridoxine-free multivitamins are available for clients taking levodopa.

a, b, and **d.** There are no contraindications to taking vitamin D, iron, and zinc for the client with Parkinson's disease who is taking levodopa. Since Mr. Arters may have trouble chewing and swallowing due to his Parkinson's disease, his intake of meats may be reduced. Thus, iron and zinc supplementation may be important.

23. **Correct answer is a.** A metallic taste is a common side effect of iodine.

    b. Large doses of iodine may cause diarrhea. Iodine does not slow peristalsis.
    c. Iodine does not cause osmotic diuresis.
    d. Fever is more likely than hypothermia to occur as a side effect of iodine.

24. **Correct answer is c.** Polymyxin B is nephrotoxic and neurotoxic. One indicator of neurotoxicity is an unsteady gait.

    a. Jaundice is a sign of hepatotoxicity, which is not a common problem with polymyxin B.
    b. Dyspnea is a sign of respiratory depression or pulmonary toxicity, neither of which is a common effect of polymyxin B.
    d. An irregular pulse is related to cardiac toxicity, which is not common with polymyxin B.

25. **Correct answer is a.** For older children and adults, pulling the pinna up and back will straighten the ear canal.

    b. Pulling the lobe of the ear down and back straightens the ear canal in children under 4.
    c. Pulling the pinna outward at a 45° angle does not straighten the ear canal.
    d. Pulling the pinna up and back is the appropriate means of administering ear medication to children 4 and older and to adults.